T0127727

Meds & Remedies

ALAIN AMZALLAG – Ph.D.

authorHOUSE®

AuthorHouse™
1663 Liberty Drive
Bloomington, IN 47403
www.authorhouse.com
Phone: 1 (800) 839-8640

Published by AuthorHouse 06/08/2018

ISBN: 978-1-5462-4003-7 (sc)
ISBN: 978-1-5462-4002-0 (e)

Library of Congress Control Number: 2018905203

Print information available on the last page.

Contents

APPENDIX
cancer

Dedication

It is with immense gratitude and appreciation that the author dedicates "Meds & Remedies" to the staff of the dialysis unit of the CHSM of MTL for the TLC they afforded to Alain A...

Nurses / technicians & Staff at the St- Mary's Hptl's Dialysis Unit

- Mary W., R.N.
- Shirley, R.N.
- Scott, R.N.
- Ken, R.N.
- Nelly, R.N.
- Mary-Lou, R.N.
- George, R.N.
- Rima, Sec.
- Elizabeth, Head R.N.
- Nadia, R.N.
- Ted, R.N.
- Christine, R.N.
- Lorraine K, R.N.
- Merrie, R.N.
- Marie, R.N.
- Mary, R.N.
- Georgia, R.N
- Hanan, R.N
- Sofia, R.N.
- Martin, R.N. Supervisor
- Arturo, R.N.
- Adelia, S. R.N.
- Howard, T. P.A.B.
- Veronica, P.A.P.
- Francois, P.A.B.
- Claudia, Hous.
- Jennifer, R.N.

Albert Einstein Quotes

"Einstein, a Jewish-American theoretical physicist advanced the field of Physics, ahead if his time" In 1905, at age 26, Einstein published:

- *The Photoelectric Effect, used Plank's Quantum Hypothesis.*
- *Special Theory of Relativity.*
- *How Mass and Energy were equivalent.*

"Albert Einstein developed also the General Theory of Relativity"

"The most beautiful thing we can experience is the mysterious. It is the source of all true art and science"

"An empty stomach is not a good political advisor"

"I never think of the future. It comes soon enough"

"When a man sits with a pretty girl for an hour, it seems like a minute. But let him sit on a hot stove for a minute – and it's longer than any hour. That's relativity"

"I think and think for months and years. Ninety-nine times, the conclusion is false. The hundredth time I am right"

"Solitude is painful when one is young, but delightful when one is more mature"

"Sometimes one pays most for the things one gets for nothing"

"Everything should be made as simple as possible, but not simpler"

"Try not to become a man of success but rather try to become a man of value"

"He who can no longer pause to wonder and stand rapt in awe is as good as dead; his eyes are closed"

"Science without religion is lame" "Religion without science is blind"

Education is that which remains when one has forgotten everything one learned in school"

"Gravity cannot be held responsible for people falling in love"

"There are two ways to live your life. One is as though nothing is a miracle. The other is as though everything is a miracle"

"Imagination is more important that knowledge"

"Only two things are infinite, the universe and human stupidity and I am not sure about the former"

Since the mathematicians have invaded the theory of relativity, I do not understand it myself anymore'

"The human mind has first to construct forms independently, before we can find them in things"

These thoughts did not come in my verbal formulation. I rarely think in words at all. A thought comes, and I may try to express it in words afterwards"

"Great spirits have always found violent opposition from mediocrities – The latter cannot understand it when a man does not thoughtlessly submit to hereditary prejudices but honestly and courageously uses his/her intelligence"

-=-=-=-=-

"When Wisdom unites with Intelligence, Complete Understanding ensues and beyond that point loss of reason is possible" – Kabbalah

-=-=-=-=-

Alain's Promise

I AM LOOKING FOR GOOD WOMAN;

- To laugh with…
- To interact harmoniously with…
- To love & cherish…
- To buffer emotions with…
- To stimulate intellectually…
- To make allowances for…
- To understand…
- To forgive easily…
- To never to give up on…
- To provide encouragement for…
- To provide comforting words to…
- To provide spiritual sustenance to…
- To be a T.L.C. provider…
- To lend a shoulder to lean on…
- To dry our respective tears…

WITH ANTICIPATED LOVE, CARING & RESPECT…

I AM WAITING FOR YOU…

Alain Amzallag, PhD (ABD)

October 2011

Montreal

A Smile

A smile costs nothing
But it has a great value
It enriches the recipient
Without impoverishing the giver

It lasts an instant
But lingers on
No one is too rich to do without
But poor people can possess it
It makes families happy
Businesses successful, friendships long lasting

A smile relaxes us
When we are tired
Encourages us
When we are depressed
Comforts us when we are sad
And helps us fight all our worries

However it cannot be bought
Borrowed or stolen
It has value
Only when it is given

If you meet someone
Who does not give you the smile
That you deserve
Be generous, give him yours
For no one needs more
A smile than someone
Who cannot give it to others

Translated from French by:
Alain Amzallag, M.Sc.
December 9th, 2005

Giving Time

POEM(E) II (F&E)   BS"D

GIVING TIME

To an Elder,
To a Child,
To a Son,
To a Daughter,
To a Friend,
To a Spouse.

GIVING TIME IS GIVING LOVE!

DONNER DU TEMPS

À un Vieillard,
À un Enfant,
À un Fils,
À une Fille,
À un Ami,
À un Époux,

DONNER DU TEMPS C'EST DONNER DE L'AMOUR!

Alain Amzallag

Le 19 Septembre, 2005

Overview

At the time of his Bar Mitzvah at age 13, Alain Amzallag acquired an intense, consuming desire to eradicate cancer once and for all.

This obsession, in fact, dictated his choice of courses and programs through his school years. That included at high school, his undergraduate study and lab work at McGill University in Montreal, as well as graduate work at New York's Cornell University's Graduate School of Medical Sciences / Sloan-Kettering Division, and Rockefeller University as a specially invited student.

The author chose science courses and university programs for one reason alone: to maximize his preparation for the task at hand, namely to find that elusive cure. As well, the author registered in several successive undergraduate Honours programs at McGill, most notably;

- From 1967-1968 – Honours Microbiology & Immunology & Virology
- From 1968-1869 – Honours Bacterial Genetics
- From 1969-1970 – Honours Molecular Genetics & Honours Biochemistry.

By doing all of the above, the author was to approach finding a cure for cancer from a wide variety of perspectives, something to give a budding, noble researcher hope for success by choosing areas of study correctly, in an organized and logical way.

In September 1971, Amzallag began his research in immunogenetics, that is, the study of cell surface components (antigens and/or receptors), using various immunological techniques and this, in various histocompatibility [(H-2) and T - Brachyury loci in mice.

As well, the author carried out a study of alloantigens using indirect immunofluorescence on lymphocytes, spermatozoa and fresh frozen cryostat sections of 1 µm in thickness. This enabled Amzallag to visualize the intra organ tissues as adjacent cells have a membrane in common.

The author saw that having a "handle" -- or rather a "slice "of the cell surface (tangentially) -- provided him with an increased awareness and visualization of the events occurring at the cell surface level in the context of topology and morphogenetic movements within tissues (lymphoid or solid). This process (differentiation) as studied in a normal mouse model was useful to understand what actually goes wrong during invasiveness, metastases as well as loss of contact inhibition. Also, the author studied alloantigens on mouse thymocytes, lymphocytes, spermatozoa in cell suspensions, and cryostat sections of mouse testes, thymus, lymph nodes, spleen, and so on.

In addition, Amzallag carried out an experiment (no data available) designed to establish and prove the presence of alleles at the H-Y and H-X loci in mice, by grafting pieces of skin from F1 hybrids (from inbred strains) onto corresponding reciprocal F1 recipients, and by then scoring rejection or tolerance of the grafts.

It is important to appreciate the fact that every strain (inbred, F1 hybrid, backcross, congenic) of mice originated from the late Gloria Thomas Alexander, R.N.'s mouse colony. She was a gifted, industrious scientist and took special orders (any reasonable number) of mice of any genotype, i.e., congenic at only one gene (allele) for example H-2 k on a Balb/c Background.

Everything was proceeding apace until the fall of 1973 when the author descended into the depths of a major clinical depression, deep enough to require medication. The medication elevated Amzallag's mood, but in the spring of 1974, something unexpected and remarkable occurred: the author had a spectacular "vision" and acute schizoid episode that required psychiatric hospitalization for six weeks. At the Payne-Whitney Clinic where he was treated, Amzallag repeated incessantly that he had "discovered a cure for cancer" and that his father was "authoritarian". At the peak of this manic episode, the author was so in touch with his own physiology that he claimed that if told the normal ranges of biochemical parameters, he could hazard an accurate guess of his own. However, this 'impression' remained unproven as during Alain's stay at the Payne-Whitney clinic, it was never tested.

At this juncture in the author's life, it became apparent that something of huge significance had occurred in his brain. It seemed that that Alain was able to conceptualize, mentally, the answer to his long sought quest: to develop a universal theoretical protocol to treat all cancers and other chronic diseases. Eventually, Alain, in 2005, wrote Theoretical and Practical Notions in Cancer Immunotherapy, which he sent to Dr Cliff Stanners of McGill University Biochemistry / Cancer Centre, and to Dr. Lawrence Panasci of the Lady Davis Institute / JGH.

In the spring of 1983, Amzallag began his position as senior Territory Sales Manager with *Canadian* Life Technologies Inc., promoting and selling scientific and medical research supplies to research and clinical laboratories in major Canadian cities (mostly in Ontario and Quebec) as well as for three years in the Maritimes and Newfoundland. In that capacity, the author travelled extensively and met regularly with hundreds of scientific personnel: undergraduate and graduate students, research assistants and associates, postdoctoral fellows and principal investigators. The discussion did not focus exclusively on the products, but also occasionally on the research their laboratory was engaged in. Occasionally, Amzallag himself had the opportunity to suggest avenues of experimentation that, when applied, resulted in positive outcomes. It felt good, he felt, to be useful scientifically once again, like old times.

The author would also like to take note, with all due humility, that his position as Senior Territory Sales Manager at *Canadian* LTI was very successful, principally because he earned great credibility, scientifically and ethically bestowing to the scientists and the clinicians the respect that is their due for the nobility of their scientific and human pusuits.

In turn, the researchers always considered Alain Amzallag a friend and a colleague, especially at McGill, his alma mater.

Biography

Born in 1949 in Casablanca, Morocco, Alain Amzallag, in the early 60's decides that he will become a scientist and sets his sights on "finding a cure for cancer". Up until 1970, Alain studies scientific and medical topics so as to prepare himself to achieve this goal. When he was 21 years old, the author entered a Ph.D. program at the Cornell University Graduate School of Medical Sciences/Sloan-Kettering Division, in Manhattan. There, he undertakes several projects in Immunogenetics with success.

Besides distractions of social nature (chess, bridge & volleyball) Alain studies hard and with determination. Following an unfortunate love betrayal, Alain slips into a major depression in the Fall of 1973. Once the depression is over, his mood is buoyant and he undertakes in the Spring of 1974 a marathon of 72 hours accompanied with sleep and food deprivation during which he works on a theoretical approach to cancer therapy. During his retreat in the dormitory room, he has a vision. This vision encompasses an integrated comprehension of the immunological aspect of cancer and other chronic diseases.

Towards the end of the vision, the author loses contact with reality and is subsequently hospitalized and diagnosed as having had an 'acute schizoid episode'. In this book, Anatomy of a vision (Fondation Littéraire Fleur de Lys), you will find the description of the prevailing mental state before, during and after the vision as well as the outlining of the vision

-=-=-=-=-

FROM BIPOLAR DISTRESS TO MY RECOVERY
BY
Alain Amzallag, Ph.D (ABD).
Montréal, Canada

In the fall of '73 I began my slide into a severe depression, deep in anguish and anxiety. The following Spring I experienced an Acute Schizoid episode.

This was my first manic episode. It presented a loss of contact with reality (psychosis) and interrupted my promising studies and work at the Cornell University Graduate School of Medical Sciences where I was in the process of conducting cancer research as a doctoral candidate.

In the Summer of '74, I presented part of my work to the Cornell University Faculty where I obtained a Master of Science degree. Although I had many obstacles to overcome at that point in my life, I remained motivated and attempted to complete my Ph.D.

The story of my recovery began in 1981. I was diagnosed with Bipolar Affective Disorder, Type 1, (Manic-Depressive Illness). Since that first depression in 1973, I have identified nine challenges that I feel are necessary to recovery.

This article will provide a testimonial as to what steps could be taken in order to start the recovery process, ultimately leading to mood stabilization and healing. The nine challenges are:

1 - To emerge intact from the steamroller of the first major depression.
2 - To wait patiently for the correct diagnosis.
3 - To accept the diagnosis after a period of denial.
4 - To gear up and decide to learn how to manage the condition.
5 - To find a Psychiatrist that you fully trust.
6 - To take your medication as directed.
7 - To eliminate drugs and alcohol completely.
8 - To adjust the doses of medications within the therapeutic window with your physician's approval.
9 - To seek support from among the following: Psychiatrists, Psychologists, Psychiatric Nurses, Social Workers, Occupational therapists, Self-esteem workshops, Mental Health Associations, Internet Chat Rooms and so on.

From 1981 to 2002, despite mood fluctuations of various intensities ranging from hypomania, irritability and depression, this period of my life was the most productive for my family and me. I was relatively functional and was able to maintain the same job for over 20 years. During this time,

I provided for my family and helped to raise four wonderful and talented children; all valuable and contributing members of society.

After my last episode in 2002, I embraced change and became an author, artist and musician. Volunteer work as a musician in seniors' residences was gratifying for me, confirming my belief that "giving of oneself without expecting returns" has its own rewards. These artistic, literary and musical endeavours helped me reach perfect Harmony within myself.

I was fortunate to connect with the Cummings Jewish Centre for Seniors Mental Health Program. Their support brought more stability and well-being into my life.

One thing is certain; in order to achieve my recovery I had to realize that I had to be the 'conductor' of my own life, my moods and attitudes, with the spirit of courage, tenacity and resilience.

My greatest desire is that the stigmas about mental illness will diminish; eventually disappearing so that mentally affected persons can seek and obtain the care and support that they need: safely, freely, openly and humanely.

(Revised by Laura Steen, Port Hope, Ontario)

-=-=-=-=-

PLEASE, CONSIDER SUPPORTING GENEROUSLY:

- La Fraternité des Policiers et des Policières de Montréal
- The War Amps
- La Fondation CHU Sainte-Justine
- La Fédération Québécoise du cancer
- The Kidney Foundation of Canada
- Société Canadienne de la Sclérose en Plaques
- Amiquebec
- Revivre
- Cancer de la Prostate Canada
- Friends of the Simon Wiesenthal Center for Holocaust Studies

Longevity & Cigarette Smoking

Based on what was established about regulatory genes and gene products in Procaryotes (operons) and subsequently in Eucaryotes (multi-genic, multifactoriel & pleiotropic loci) as well as some empirical observations by Alain A., A.A.A. is comfortable stating that hereditary and genetic transmission of genes insuring longevity will prevail at medium and long terms over the cancer inducing effect of carcinogenic (mutation causing) chemicals present in cigarette tar.

The corollary of this statement is that A.A.A. has decided that he will no longer attempt to quit smoking as he believes his 49 years of heavy smoking is congruent with the notion described above that quitting suddenly might just induce cancer.

Alain A. feels the above is neither a rationalization nor a justification to continue smoking as several individuals who smoked all their lives lived to be healthy and kicking in their ninety's - G-d bless them. This observation is in contradistinction with the fact that even though they have not smoked a single cigarette, some persons have developed lung cancer.

As added bonus which hopefully will playa role in the duration of A.A.A.'s life is the fact that all his male ancestors on his father side lived well over their nineties.

So, at least with a small sample, it would seem that there is an indication that smoking is safe for Alain and may Ie Lord grant him a long Life in Health... BS"D.

Urination

"Even if you shake it, the last drop will go into your pants" – Graffiti on bathroom wall at Northmount High School (1965)

As old age takes its toll, it becomes more and more strenuous to generate a smooth and constant flow of urine. However, with an ultimate effort, a pleasant surprise may occur, namely; "a brief orgasmic piss burst".

<u>Thermo-reflex</u>: Urologist Keith Mathews, M.D., of Cardiogenix agreed with A.A.A. that the efficient voiding of the bladder by putting <u>cold tap water</u> on fingers or hand while urinating is indeed an example of thermo-reflex. This empirical observation that this trick will increase the flow and the output (total volume) of urine eliminated was confirmed by Dr. Matthews to be real and represented a clever way to achieve the desired result; namely, controlling partial or total incontinence (bed wetting).

<u>Self massage</u>:

In addition to thermo-reflex, massaging one's own urethra, firmly yet gently, will most likely accelerate and contribute to the total voiding of the bladder. This is important before weighing oneself before dialysis and after dialysis so as to establish an accurate and precise weight gain or loss as a result of the treatment.

In general, the patient must void completely his/her bladder before he <u>weighs</u> him/herself prior to being hooked up with the dialysis apparatus. Following the <u>dialysis</u> treatment, the patient weighs him or herself one more in order to establish the gain / loss of liquid as a result of the treatment.

The gradual and the total weight loss is a function of the seriousness with which the transplant candidate follows his/her assigned severe renal diet as well as the duration and the frequency of the dialysis treatments.

It goes without saying that weight loss and thinning of the body renders the perspective recipient healthier and readier to receive a kidney graft and renders the whole procedure of getting ready to receive this "gift of a renewed and improved life" very much impregnated with hope and anticipation of a forthcoming gratitude to my three Nephrologists, Paul Bourgoin, M.D.; Natalie Ng Cheong, M.D. & Dre. Eid., M.D.

The team of nurses / technicians composed of devoted individuals with a kind heart and huge skills make the 'ordeal' of being dialysed almost an activity to look forward to, i. e., always smiling and vigilant in case should an emergency occurs. If and that that happens, they are extremely quick to respond and reinstate order in the Dialysis Unit and normalcy to the process which, by all accounts, is harmonious and proceeds always with the spirit of cooperation and collaboration between the unit's staff. "May Allah, the Lord and Hashem" grant them a long life in health so that they be able to continue to excel in their blessed endeavour, namely; alleviate suffering and prolong the life of patients whom, some of us are, in a terminal status.

Alain A.'S Diet Items

GLUCIDES: 1 sachet de sucre = 1c. thé = 5 glucides. (Carbohydrates).

A) 4 portions (at least) of vegetables (5 gms de glucides)
- 1 cup of vegetable raw- ½ cup of vegetable cooked.
- 1 x 25 ml de jus de légumes. Green vegetables mostly.

B) 2-5 portions par jour... 15 large grapes = 1 portion
- 1 cup of water melon, strawberries, raspsberries, blueberries

PROTEINS : -7 gm Proteins = 1 once of meat-chiken-fish

Aim for 80 GMS OF PROTEIN PER DAY

- 2 portions de protéine par jour; 35+35+ 2-3 gm / tr. de pain.

MILK PRODUCTS: 2-4 portions daily- 1 Cup of milk (250 ml) = 1 portion

- -3/4 cup of yogurt = 1 portion

STARTCHES (AMIDON) 6-10 portions /day

NO = ZERO: Trans-fat; zero saturated fats...

FATS: - (Gras) 1c à thé of Canola oil (5ml) 4-8 per day.

- Only unsaturated fats (Triglycerides)
- 1/6 of Avocado = 1 portion of fat

NOTE : I am truly greateful to Mrs. Nicole Sabourin, Dietician for the knowledge of the components of the prescribed renal diet she imparted to me... Also, the actual Dietetician of the Nephrology Department of the st.Mary's Hospital, Natalia, is doing a great job in helping me to hone the renal diet I am following stritly.

Kidney Function & Dialysis

Kidney function is paramount for survival. The complete loss of kidney function is terminal, and death ensues. To maintain and sustain life, a kidney transplant from a live or deceased donor is required. Until such a kidney is available, dialysis provides a way to affect the usual functions of this organ namely; removal of excess liquid, detoxication of the blood, and so on.

Together with dialysis, some exercise to strengthen muscles and other organs is recommended together with a severe renal diet. Part and parcel of the renal diet for chronic diseased kidney patients is the oft-prescribed liquid restriction. Indeed, the dialysis apparatus replaces the removal of excess fluids which a normal healthy kidney does. During his dialysis treatments, the author was limited to 1,5 liters of liquid per day. Everything contributes to this 1,5-liter restriction; even the H2O absorbed during swallowing of medications; it is an accounting nightmare. But, it must be done!

About liquid input limit, drink in small gulps, few and far between helps with side effects such as a dry mouth. The uptake of some medications and some foods leads to intense thirst. In such cases, candies without added sugar can possibly yield additional salivation.

Weight Variation

To prepare Alain A.'s body to receive a kidney transplant to increase his renal function of filtering liquids (blood, urine, and so on.) dialysis and a severe renal diet were prescribed and started simultaneously on November 6th, 2016.

The observed consequences of this serious commitment to dialysis and renal diet are:

- Loss of weight was observed during the duration of the dialysis treatments (three sessions of four hours per week) is congruent with the conclusion that Alain A.'s body was getting healthier.
- An increased level of energy became evident as the procedures were carried out and the strengthening of Alain's limbs were concomitant with the start of dialysis, i.e., November 2016.
- His weight in October 2016 was 249 lbs / 113 kgs and on November 2017 the weight was: 211,2lbs / 96.0 kgs This amounts to a total loss of 37,8 lbs / 17 kgs during treatments over one year.

P.S., Please, see chapter on Urination for more info about dialysis & weight variation... Thanks.

The Dialysis Effect On Alain Amzallag

Great news:

Prior to dialysis on Feb. 2, 2017:
- Glucose: 7.9 mmol/ L
- Urea: 27.6 mmol/ L
- Creatine: 695 µmole/ L
- Magnesium: 1.07 mmol/ L
- Albumin: 34 g/ L

After dialysis on Feb. 2, 2017:
- Urea: 10.5 mmole/ L
- Creatine: 329 µmole / L
- Hb: 111 g/ L
- Ferritin: 19 µg / L
- Iron: 8 µmole / L

Post-dialysis (Feb. 25, 2017):
- Hb 101g/ L

The author's daily medications
(February, 2017)

6 AM (upon waking)
- Pantolac (40 mg))

8 AM (breakfast)
- Colace (2 gelcaps)
- Epival (750 mg)
- Orap (4 mg)
- Furosemide (80 mg)
- Vitamin D (3,000 U.I.)
- Vitalux (Eye health)
- Forsenol (1,000 mg) (to maintain normal levels of Phosphorus)

NOON (lunch)
- Calcium (500 mg)
- Replavite (?)
- Forsenol (1,000 mg)

6 PM (supper)
- Epival (750 mg)
- Colace (2 gelules)
- Norvask (5 mg)
- Furosemide (80 mg)
- Forsenol (1,000 mg)

11 PM (bedtime)
- Seroquel (400 mg)
- Lipitor (10 mg)

The author's daily medications
in March, 2017

6 AM
- Pantelac (40 MG)

8 AM
- Colace (2 gelules)
- Epival (750 mg)
- Furosémide (80 mg)
- Vitamine D (3,000 U.I.)
- Vitalux (santé des yeux)

NOON:
- Calcium (500 mg)
- Replavite (?)

6 PM
- Epival (750 mg)
- Colace (2 gelules)
- Norvask (5 mg)
- Furosémide (80 mg)

11 PM
- Seroquel (400 mg)
- Lipitor (10 MG)

Alain Amzallag – Ph.D.

Maple syrup facilitates the efficacy of antibiotics in fighting bacterial infections.

Indigenous peoples have long known that maple syrup has healing properties. Fewer antibiotics, for example, will be needed to kill off the bacteria because the cell wall of the microorganism is weakened by maple syrup, allowing the antibiotic to more readily enter the cytoplasm of the microbe and more efficiently kill it. In this fashion, I am certain, maple syrup will play a major role in counteracting the increase in antibiotic resistance due to overuse being observed in every aspect of our lives.

The author's medications
in October, 2017

6 AM Pantolac (40 mg) – Coats & protects stomach

8 AM Colace (two gelcaps) – for constipation
Vitamin D (3,000 U.I.) [Protection against cancer]

Renvela 800 mg – Lowers and maintains stable phosphorus.
Lasix (160 mg) (Furosemide) Increases urination and reduces edema.
Abilify (20 mg) – Anti psychotic.

NOON
Calcium (500 mg) Calcification – Absorption of Vitamin D
- Renvela (800 mg) – Lowers Phosphorus level

6 PM
Colace (2 gelules) - Constipation
Norvask (5 mg) - for hypertension - To be taken after dialysis
treatment as per Dr. Johanna Eid.
Renvela (800 mg) – lowers phosphorus level

11 PM
- Seroquel - (Quetiapine)(400 mg) (Anti psychotic) + sedative effect
- Epival – (Valproic acid) - 1500 mg (Anti psychotic)
- Lipitor (10 mg) - Lowers Cholesterol

Note: The author has observed empirically that the taking of medication
should be routine: at the same fixed times in respect to meals and snacks.
This is beneficial to the physiological homeostasis of the individual.

Neurotransmitters

The foods we eat are converted into sub-units through the process of catabolism and are then used to synthesize (during anabolism) into larger molecules that function within the brain. These molecules -- called neurotransmitters -- control several aspects of mood and energy levels.

NEUROTRANSMITTERS:

Under the general heading of *Mood Stabilizers*, the following is a presentation based on an article by Isabelle Artus – with sections summarized by Didier Chos -- on how nutritional elements help regulate variations in mood.

"Dopamine, Serotonin and Noradrenalin are neurotransmitters that together regulate mood, energy level, and our sense of harmoniousness – in other words, how happy we feel. When the level of serotonin is insufficient, the mood dips quickly, sometimes causing aggressiveness. this is followed by sleep disorders, bad mood and sometimes depression. Serotonin is labeled the "Good Humor Hormone." The amino acid tryptophan -- a precursor to serotonin and dopamine -- and craving foods that contain Tryptophan -- are necessary to maintain a stable level of these two neurotransmitters. Starchy foods, fish, rice etc. all contain Tryptophan. However, too many simple sugars, and/or stimulants like nicotine or caffeine, reduce the level of serotonin in the brain because your system depletes your serotonin reserve as you metabolize these substances. You might ingest these substances and feel a "high," but that mood crashes a few hours later, perpetuating the addiction cycle.

It has long been established in the medical community that a large number of the same medications (pills or other…) can be lethal. In contrast, a large number of diverse medications treating different ailments appear relatively safe!

A REMINDER: balanced blood sugars levels foster a balanced mood. To achieve that, you need sufficient serotonin-producing protein and insulin-balancing polyunsaturated "good" fats.

Now, "a deficiency in dopamine leads to difficulties in concentration and to a loss in motivation. Dopamine stimulates the heart and general metabolism. Noradrenalin increases motivation and energy levels and acts as an antidepressant. A non-essential amino acid called L-Tyrosine -- found in seafood, cheese, milk and eggs – is a precursor to noradrenalin and dopamine and facilitates adequate energy levels and a good dose of optimism -- which is why the afore mentioned foods should be eaten.

WARNING: It is of paramount importance for the reader to realize that these guidelines cannot replace prescribed medications, but they can enhance their efficacy.

Many medications -- such as mood stabilizers (Tegretol, Epival, Lamictal, Lithium Carbonate, etc.) have side effects and, having had my share of them, I can vouch that such side effects are temporary since the body and the brain acclimatize to them, and they become irrelevant. However, long-term use of Lithium carbonate (Carbolith, Lithane and Duralith), can cause irreversible damage to the thyroid gland, the kidneys and other organs. Therefore, regular monitoring of Lithium levels is essential. This ensures that the **optimal** amount of lithium is administered, while minimizing its destructive potential.

A Case in point: the author was prescribed Lithium carbonate from 1979 to 2009 for treating the symptoms of Bipolarity, type 1. This duration of treatment (30 years) proved excessive. In 2009 the author was diagnosed with chronic kidney disease. This renal insufficiency was confirmed by biopsy at the Jewish General Hospital. The pathology of the disease showed destruction of more than 80% of the glumeronephrons. The diagnosis also marked the first time the author was advised of the necessity to follow a strict renal diet, with dialysis imminent.

After eight years of despair and apprehension in anticipation of the possibility of having not to smoke, the author reviewed the test results of serum levels going back several years and understood how the lapse in vigilance could have occurred. Kidney function is monitored through the levels (μmoles per liter) of creatinine. A "normal" creatinine level is from from 40 – 126 μmoles per liter, and it is only outside this range that a low and/or a high value is flagged. It is my contention that psychiatrists and physicians look at the "red flags" instead of the 'High/Normal" values which, in retrospect, would have been the right time to stop prescribing Lithium in favor of another mood stabilizer.

NEUROLEPTICS: Moditen, Largarctil, Orap, Zyprexa.

Neuroleptics slow down the electrochemical impulses between neurons at the synaptic level. The neuroleptic Orap has been taken by the author for more than 26 years -- until March 6, 2017. At that time, he changed dosage on his own based on previous empirical observation and stopped taking the 2mg of Orap in the morning. This change -- coupled with a stopping dialysis treatment -- caused a trip to the emergency room due to a fall that rendered the author unconscious.

In general, the author was served well by Orap, since it worked well as a dampening tool for his hypomania. As soon as he felt euphoria, marked by an increased appreciation of beauty in nature, objects, music art, he -- with his psychiatrist's authorization --increased the dose of Orap to 3. 4 mg depending on the need. The upper limit, never to be exceeded, is 10 mg Orap per day. In this way, the author avoided hospitalization for 21 years -- from 1981 to 2002 – a remarkable achievement for anyone who is affected by Bipolarity, type 1. This technique of tweaking the neuroleptic (which is also a psychotropic) dose on constant and observation of one's mood, stabiized his euphoric state and general state of mental well-being.

It must be remembered that it is vital to continue taking medication until the end of the period prescribed by the psychiatrist, especially in the case of treatment of mania or the alleviation of clinical depression. It is important to never reduce the dose or the length of treatment without the physician's authorization.

Relief From Pain

The author believes that neuromuscular pain occurs mostly in limbs, bones, joints, the neck and elsewhere. The author also believes that humidity and extreme cold can worsen osteoarthritis and arthritic pain, mostly in joints. However, a natural product suggested by a physician to the author helped alleviate his joint pain from arthrosis. Called Glucosamine and Chondroitin (900 mg), the products's optimal dose is determined gradually, by starting with one pill a day followed by empirical evaluation for a month. If needed, the dosage can be increased to two and later to even three pills. The pharmacist should be consulted if no substantial decrease in pain is seen.

In general, pain can be relieved by creating or applying warmth and heat to the injured area (the author will summarize methods he first learned as a 13-year-old boy scout in Morocco). Developing a taste for healing his own self and others led the author, ultimately, to advanced studies in scientific and medical toward his main quest: to "end cancer." (please read Overview Section as well as APPENDIX CANCER).

BACK PAIN:

Often, upon awakwing in the morning the author suffers excruciating pain in the lower back (lumbar area), making it difficult to sit up or stand. One of the ways the author deals with this is to sit at the edge of the bed or seat while keeping his back as rigid as possible. At this point, pain is practically nonexistent. Next, the author moves his torso incrementally in different directions, very slowly and very carefully so as not to trigger pain. This technique is akin to a stretching exercise that warms up ligaments and the tendons in the spinal cord. This exercise, after a while, can be gradually elaborated upon, for example, by reaching over the coffee table to grab a cigarette (at least in my case). A crucial step in minimizing back pain is to use a walker or a quadruped cane to carefully stand up with one's back very straight while making sure you don't feel pain. The next thing to do is to take small steps with a straightened back and to start walking, to warm up the muscles, especially in the lower (lumbar) back area. These steps can bring the individual successfully to fulfill his morning ablutions, to use the toilet, to put on his/her socks and shoes, to get dressed, to prepare breakfast, and so on.

NECK PAIN:

Before you hire a massage therapist for neck pain, the author suggests that homework be done first. The neck is a very delicate region of the body and if handled wrongly could have dire consequences. The most important thing to do is verify the degrees and bona fides of the therapists you approach. The massage therapist should have a very solid reputation. The author was fortunate to have encountered a therapist with magic hands as Rozella puts her heart and soul to the task at hand.

ELECTRIC HOT PAD:

Please take note: _The recommended rate of usage is 20 minutes every 2 hours at low or medium setting_. Anything higher could damage the soft tissue of the area where the pad is applied. A bonus in using a heating pad is pad is that it can be applied onto practically every ailing area (including limbs) because it can be secured with elastic bandages.

Varia

Analgesics:

Tylenol, generically known as Acetaminophen, can be useful in treating headaches and generating an overall sense of well-being. It is important, though, not to consume too much, since it can potentially damage the liver. In combination with valproic acid (Epival), damage to the liver is cumulative and can result in a serious impairment of hepatic function.

Constipation:

Lax-A-Day is nowadays the preferred laxative physicians prescribe, as it is slow yet effective. Carter pills and its generic, bisacodyl, is a also a rather neat way to trigger the evacuation of the intestines. Drinking a large quantity of very chilled water at the right time can induce defecation. Other means include glycerin suppositories, enemas (which work really well but is a messy procedure and not recommended for patients with kidney problems), senna Senokot, pears, prunes, etc. If you tend to be constipated, try to minimize the daily use of dairy products.

Flatulence:

Flatulence will occur in lactose intolerant individuals who consume dairy products in liquid form. It is also advisable to avoid soft cheeses such as Brie and Camembert, and in some cases, yogurt. Flatulence is also common in individuals undergoing dialysis, when the the whole physiology of patients is in turmoil, with the intestines and rectum expanding with gasses until expelled.

Diabetes:

Measuring one's glucose level three times a day just prior to meals is essential for diabetics. Be on the lookout for hypoglycemia. If hypoglycemic, you can try to raise blood blood sugar quickly by consuming a small to moderate amount of juice or candy without added sugar. To protect against hyperglycemia, diabetic patients are sometimes prescribed Gluconorm or are injected with insulin in cases of elevated blood glucose levels.

In 2017, the author was diagnosed with minimal (type II) diabetes, which requires him to vigilantly monitor the amount of carbohydrates he takes in from prepared foods and beverages. One should remember, however, that glucose crosses the blood-brain barrier and literally provides "food for thought," an appropriate metaphor for every biochemical and neuro-physiological interaction taking place in the brain.

-=-=-=-=-

Maimonides

Rabbi Moses ben Maimon, a towering 12th century rabbi, physician and philosopher known as The Rambam (Maimonides), was instrumental in developing, to a considerable extent, fundamental principles of nutrition and medicine -- even the therapeutic use of plants and herbs. He was also a pre-eminent Torah scholar. His works, until today, are celebrated, and have affected a great part of the western world in terms of how it developed basic principles of law, medicine, science, and nutrition.

Maimonides, for example, advocated eating one slice of bread every morning so as to promote a smooth and positive healthy day. He encouraged a half-hour walk after meals, and recommended eating raw and cold foods for lunch and cooked, and warm foods for supper, so scholars and intellectuals would not get sleepy in the afternoon while they tried to focus on their studies.

Maimonides' pieces of judicious advice go on and on.

As a testament to his enduring legacy, Jewish medical students take the Oath of Maimonides when graduating, while non-Jewish medical students recite the Hippocratic Oath.

Words To The Wise

- "Victory is reached by an accumulation of small advantages."

--Chess lingo.

- "A partial victory is still a victory."
- "Revel in complexity and eschew complications."

-- The author

- "Life is as wonderful as you want it to be."

--- Kabbalah

- "Everything that happens to us is for our own good'.

--- the Zohar

- "Wisdom and discernment combine, and yield understanding."

---- Ram'hal

- "Mental health issues affect us -- but do not possess us."

-- The author

- "Being ethical is more important that legality"

--- The author

Faith

Faith is an essential component of psychological health.

Indeed, it assures survival to whoever possesses or searches for it…

The greatest punishment that the Creator could inflict upon His flock would be to deprive them or strip them of Faith…

Because without our Faith, we no longer have benchmarks, and we would be estranged from our roots and would succumb to our vain tendencies…

The so-called "religious fanatics" follow an erroneous path in their super-elevated faith, which in reality is only a proclivity for intolerance and self-destruction. Their acts show they have lost their bearings.

Those who possess true faith and have experienced telepathy with their kin know that faith represents the peaceful inner serenity of the soul…

Those who doubt the existence of G-d often expose themselves to a morose and unstable existence, susceptible to the inner corruption of parts of their soul…

BELIEF: PERCEPTION & DIVINE PRESENCE

"The voice originating from our souls expresses and resonates the wonder felt in front of the inherent beauty in everyone and everything."

"Moreover, the artistic, musical and poetic harmonies generated by innate talent developed to a maximum allows Divine creation to bask in its glorious sanctification"

Je T'aime ----- I Love You

Obitchamté (Bulgare)

Ani (m) Ohèv Otakh (f) (Hébreu)
Ani (f) Ohévet Otkha (m)
(Moderne)

Ya Tiébia Loublou (Russe)

Sarapo (Grec)

Ti Amo (Italien)

Tan 'Habak (Judéo-arabe)

Té Yubesk (Roumain)

Jeg Elsker Deg (Norvégien)

Jeg Elskar Dei (Suédois)

'nbritk (Arabe Dialectal
'Nchoffek Nord-Africain)

Dostat Doram (Afgan)

Kézi Gu Sirème (Arménien)

Toï Men Ban (Vietnamien)

Mimi Na Panda Vévé (Swahili)

Ich Liebe dich (Allemand)

Séni Sévioroum (Turc)

Yo Té Quiéro (Espagnol)

Té Amo (Latin)

Wo Aï Ni (Chinois)

Éu Gosto Déti (Portugais)

Ik Haou Van Jei (Hollandais)

Bé'Hébak (Arabe Libanais)

Ou'Hibouki(a)(Arabe Classique)

Douset Daram (Perse)
Ashghat Hastam (Perse)

Né 'Habak (Arabe Algérien)

Dama La Bëgg (Wolof-Côte
d'ivoire)

On His Way To The Mikvah

In the spring 1995, the year of the Quebec sovereignty referendum, a funny thing happened to my brother-in-law and me. Josh, then 17, was hired to "kosherize" our three-bedroom upper duplex apartment for Passover. It was established that he would get paid for the work, and the back-breaking, grueling job took Josh two and a half days to complete.

As the first seder on Passover eve fast approached, Josh needed to go to the mikvah, and as we were waiting near the 161 bus stop, he proclaimed that his hard work would be his gift to us for Passover. He was adamant about it. I vocally objected, part of me upset over his reneging that he'd get paid but the other part of me admiring his virtuous generosity.

Josh is a chassid and I am one and a half times his size. I grabbed the lapels of his traditional long black coat and gently shook him around and in mock anger, insisting he take the money.

Suddenly, the 161 bus appeared out of nowhere, the breaks slammed on, the doors flung open, and the short, portly, middle-aged bus driver leaped out and sprinted towards Josh and me shouting, to me, "Leave him alone, leave him alone!" Josh and I cracked up laughing and quickly cleared up the misunderstanding.

I find this anecdote to be invaluable for two reasons:

First, during those turbulent times of the Quebec referendum, there was at least one portly Québécois (and I am sure that there were countless others) who would stand up for the well-being of a chassidic Jew even though he could have been at risk of harm to himself.

Second, it illustrates that the social conscience of Canadians is still alive after 300-400 years.

Alain Amzallag – Ph.D.

Thus, I can say with gratitude, admiration and a sense of belonging, that:

"Il fait bon vivre au Québec"

« Canada is a great country to live in »

September 26th, 2005
(Alain Amzallag, M.Sc.)

On Top Of Ol' Cedar

There are trees, and then there are trees. The states of California and Oregon have Redwoods and the Middle East, Cypress and Cedar trees abound.

Once upon a summer vacation, my family stayed at the "Villa of Lilacs" in Ifrane, Morocco. Ifrane is a lovely village on the slopes of the Atlas range of mountains. The Atlas Mountains are majestic, and partly covered for eternity by snow.

I was four years old with a strong predilection for climbing trees, the taller the better and the more tempting to clamber up. That summer morning I was drawn to a 300 foot cedar tree and, my mother Z"L, distracted for a moment, did not see me start my climb. Like a sure-footed chimpanzee, I reached the top in no time becausae the branches were perpendicular to the trunk. After I reached the top, I sat down on a branch and feasted on the glorious scenery before me.

But because my mother did not see me, she became frantic and was sure I had been kidnapped, so she summoned the police and emergency services.

I, on the other hand, stayed serene in my contemplative location and state. At one point, looking down I noticed tiny people running around in panic. Then I decided to start my descent, again with a sure foot.

As I appeared, my mother Z"L sobbed with relief, grabbed me, hugged me and smothered me with kisses and tears. My father scolded me…

I still admire the glory of tall trees, and still have the urge to climb them, if only through imagination…

Thank you

Alain Amzallag

December 15th, 2006

To Write Or Not To Be

Expression is pleiotropic...
Verbal, facial, gestural, artistic
As with the written word.

A catharsis, a liberation or a soothing process,
Writing brings the past and the future right up to the present.

Writing enriches the author by clarifying
And simplifying the complexity of thought.
Writing brings a precise and accurate descriptive name
To what the authors imagine and feel.

Writing enables authors
To explore the unknown
Recesses of their inner voices,
And to offer their conclusions to their readers.

For the shy, without the opportunity
To express themselves otherwise, writing has become
An essential way to decipher and communicate to others
And to themselves, their most intimate and precious "jewels."

Alain Amzallag, M.Sc,
November, 2007

Appendix

A) cancer

General Theory Of cancer Management

Alain Amzallag, Ph.D. (ABD) Montréal, Canada

Statement of translational relevance

This article offers a strategy and tactics to combat cancer (in general) for review and for use by clinical cancer research professionals. It advocates initiating a multi-pronged approach with low levels of therapeutic tools; namely, the simultaneous use of chemo, radio, hormonal and/or immunological treatments at the onset of cancer therapy. These low levels are to be followed, according to the author, by several intermediary doses to finally reach an optimal therapeutic level. Each increase is done in discrete steps and is monitored for the gradual retreat of cancer. Flexibility is inherent for the oncologist as he (or she) has substantial margins in which to select and adjust the doses of therapeutic agents and techniques.

Abstract

In the midst of cancer research and work at Cornell University Graduate School of Medical Sciences / Sloan-Kettering Division, the author conceptualized, in 1974, the *"Systems Equilibrium Theory as a General Theory of Cancer Management"*. The two theories come with protocols of various therapies which are inherently flexible in nature and are 'made to measure' for each cancer patient and the effect of which are to be monitored as the strategies and tactics unfold. The protocol is, for all intents and purposes, an aggressive multi-***pronged*** attack on cancer, initially with low doses of therapeutic agent(s) and gradually, in discrete steps, followed by increased levels of anti cancer therapies up until an optimal level is reached. In this fashion, healthy cell and tissues will be spared and cancer cells and tissues will be exposed to the ***synergetic*** effects of several types of treatments. Once the patient is 'cancer free', the author advocates a maintenance dose of low level of therapeutic agent(s) to help preclude a recurrence of cancer. Moreover, appropriate diet, exercise and taking a daily 'cocktail of antioxidants' is recommended by the author to catalyze a thorough **_return to health_**.

The mainstay of the *General theory of cancer management* resides in using small simultaneous doses of the therapeutic agents and tools — Chemotherapy, radiotherapy and/or hormonal therapy —at the onset of the treatment, and then in gradually increasing the doses while monitoring their effects on the cancer. For every individual, for every type of cancer and for every stage in the development of the cancer, it seems to the author that there exists an optimal level of made-to-measure anti-cancer actions in a **multi-pronged** approach, which needs to be carried out. "Optimal" refers to the concept of targeting the treatment(s) at the cancer and sparing, as much as possible, the healthy cells making up the body's tissues and organs. If and when health is restored, as a complete concomitant remission may follow, there needs to be a continued minimal, yet essential, level of preventive treatment in order to preclude a cancer relapse in the individual.

cancer therapy

After cancer detection, the general practitioner and the clinical oncologist determine the protocols to be used on the patient in order to eradicate the cancer. These decisions have to be taken in conjunction with pre-existing medical conditions:

1) It is important to establish the duration of the first phase of treatment.
2) In each phase, the types of treatments (chemo, radio, hormonal and immunological) are to be used **simultaneously**.
3) The cancer has to be aggressively combated using a multi-pronged approach starting at very small doses of treatment together, progressively increasing the doses during intermediary stages while monitoring the effects of the treatment on the cancer cells and/ or tissues.

4) Over several stages of **incremental small increases** of the treatment, flexibility is in order as the oncologist can decide whether to favor at any given point in time a type of therapy over another based on his/her experience.

5) The patient should attempt to acquire a healthy mind (mental health, morale) and a healthy body (via physical exercise and walking, among other things).

6) Equally beneficial to some people is to rely on a spiritual practice, i.e. to pray to a higher power... asking It to spare you this time around, by guiding the mind and the hand of your oncologist.

7) Most importantly, a message for cancer patients; Do not give up on yourself – keep hoping for a return to health, no matter what! Also, the fact that nowadays, in 2009, to the author's knowledge, approximately 50% of all cancers are treated successfully should instill some hope and prompt the patient to seek bio-psycho-social help as needed. This type of support is available in medical institutions; physicians, nurses, psychologists, social workers, occupational therapists, music therapists, laughter workshops, and so on. Family and friends can also be a mainstay in providing support.

A notion arising from chess strategy was instrumental in influencing the development of the *General theory of Cancer Management*. At the start of a Chess game, the two players are on a level playing field and as the game progresses, the different moves of the pieces result in slightly improving the positional or material gains and advantages for one of the two players. When one side progresses forward, the other loses ground proportionately. If pursued, this course of action leads to the victory by one side over the other; hence the saying: "Victory is an accumulation of small advantages." In cancer management, cancer is on one side of the chessboard and the patient, with the care of the oncologist, is on the opposite side. Little by little, the patient increases his strengths—general health, strong immunity, appropriate nutrition, optimistic morale, good physical shape, etc.—at the same time using *small doses of anti-cancer therapies*, in a *protracted fashion*, and increasing them gradually as the cancer loosens its grip on the patient. This strategy will, according to the author, result in the gradual restoration of the homeostatic (*Systems*) equilibrium. Keeping in mind that the cancer patient is undertaking the fight *of* his or her life and *for* his or her life, there is always hope and desire to return to normalcy! And it is crucial to look for and revel in small improvements.

Theoretical and practical notions in cancer immunotherapy[1] (1974) (2000) (2010) (2005) (2014)

In the early 1970's, a prevalent theory about cancer postulated that cancer is an imbalance of the homeostasis of the organism. The author believes this is still largely true. Indeed, the exposure to radiation, chemical mutagens, or oncogenic viruses will result in the accumulation of mutations in the DNA sequence and cancer will ensue. If the DNA repair and later the immune surveillance mechanisms are not able to cope with these mutations past a genetically predetermined threshold, cancer will occur. The mechanism by which the loss of contact inhibition, invasiveness and metastasis operates is at the cell surface level. Cell membrane surface components mediate morphogenesis in tissues of healthy organisms. In cancer, growth occurs beyond the normal limits, with morphogenesis gone awry. In practical terms, a currently untested approach to attempt to treat cancer would be to expose cryptic cell surface tumor specific antigens derived from cancer cells or tissues by a variety of mechanical or enzymatic digestion techniques including cutting into small pieces (mincing), fragmenting with sound waves (sonicating) or enzymatically using pepsin or papain in dissociating the tumor cell membrane, while ensuring that the antigenic determinants such as Glycoproteins are not modified, altered or have lost their secondary structure. Then, the resulting preparation would be mixed with adjuvant and administered to the patient. Presumably, the antigenic determinants, previously cryptic, in this self-originating vaccine would have become immunogenic, and elicit an immune response directed towards the tumor-specific antigens of the cancer cells or tissues. In this fashion, the homeostatic equilibrium would be restored and would be concomitant with a return to health.

"We have to beat cancer, all of us, together"

Terry Fox

References:

1 This section is reprinted from Amzallag Alain © 2005, *"High, Flat, Down and Back Up Again!""A Guide to Manic-Depressive Illness"*. AuthorHouse, Bloomington, IN: 2005, pages 107-110.

Amzallag Alain © 2009 « Anatomy of a vision » « Systems Equilibrium Theory as a general Theory of Cancer Management » Fondation littéraire Fleur de Lys, Lévis, Québec G6V 2L1, Canada www.manuscritdepot.com

Amzallag Alain © 2009 « Bipolarité et Cancérologie » « Défis et Espoirs » Fondation Littéraire Fleur de Lys, Lévis, Québec G6V 2L1, Canada www.manuscritdepot.com

Addendum I

Outline Of A Vision

In the spring of 1974, during a manic episode of Bipolarity, Type 1, the author perceived a revolutionary method to treat cancer and other chronic diseases. This method which is comprised of a unifying strategy and tactics has since then been used as a springboard for several research and clinical endeavours with excellent results.

Firstly, this "General Theory of Cancer Management and other Chronic Diseases" is based on protocols of chemotherapy, radiotherapy, hormone therapy and immunotherapy (singly or combined) which proceed by a progressive and incremental increase of doses of treatments. Indeed, the level and the intensity of these treatments augment in discrete stages; first at a low dose, then at several succeeding intermediary doses, and finally at an "optimal therapeutic level", which take into account the sensitivity and the specificity of the cancer as well as that of the therapeutic tool.

Once the malignant tumor has been eliminated by standards and criteria dictated by the oncologist who follows the treatment, a slight maintenance dose of the therap(ies)y used would be advantageous and advisable to perform as it would reduce the risk of a recurrence of the cancer. Indeed, the total elimination of cancer in the patient is contingent upon insuring that no cancerous cells remain in the organism. However, this degree of certainty depends on the sensitivity and the specificity of the technique used for the detection of very few cancer cells, as a single cancer cell could theoretically repopulate the body with neoplasia. This is why a minimal maintenance dose of anti-cancer agents is primordial in order to maintain "homeostasis".

This low maintenance dose would support and assist the cellular "DNA repair" and the "Immune surveillance" systems as these two mechanisms would help "preclude" the resurgence of malignancy.

The notion of gradually restoring the "Systemic equilibrium" without upsetting the proper functioning of the patient's body has valid and therapeutic value.

Systemic equilibrium:

"This notion of systemic equilibrium was accompanied by the following defining methodology. The author thought it important to confront the noxious element (the Cancer) with chemo, radiological, hormonal and immunotherapy in increasing doses at the same time as one increases the health of other party, i.e. the body. The immune system has to be boosted in parallel with the patient's general well-being. This would comprise vitamins and minerals to be administered if deficiencies are detected and physical exercise to increase vigour and well-being. The idea is to decrease the presence, the effect and the spread of the cancer and at the same time to stimulate the body to fight back against the cancer. In this way, "homeostatic equilibrium" will be restored".

Reprinted from: 2005 – "High, Flat, Down And Back Up Again" 'A Guide to Manic-Depressive Illness' Alain Amzallag, M.Sc.. AuthorHouse, Bloomington, IN 47403. www.authorhouse.com/bookstore. page 62

"Theoretical and practical notions in cancer immunotherapy:

Written November 20th, 2000 (1974)

In the early 1970's, a prevalent theory about cancer postulated that it is an imbalance of the homeostasis of the organism. The author still believes this is largely true. Indeed, the exposure to radiation, chemical mutagens and/ or oncogenic viruses will result in the accumulation of mutations in the DNA sequence (oncogenes) and neoplasia will ensue. If DNA Repair and later the immune surveillance mechanisms are not able to cope with these mutations past a genetically predetermined threshold, cancer will occur.

Alain Amzallag – Ph.D.

The mechanism by which the loss of contact inhibition, invasiveness and metastasia operate is at the cell surface level. Cell membrane surface components mediate morphogenetic movement in tissues of healthy organisms and this cell movement goes awry in cancer.

In practical terms an as yet untested approach to attempt to treat cancer would be to expose cell surface tumor specific antigens from cancer cells or tissues by a variety of mechanical techniques including mincing, sonicating and/or slow and partial enzyme mediated dissociation, etc…. of the tumor cell membrane, while ensuring that the antigenic determinants such as glycoproteins are not modified, altered or denatured.Then the emulsion (adjuvant?) would be administered to the patient and presumably the antigenic determinants in the self originating vaccine would have become immunogenic and would elicit an immune response directed towards the tumor specific antigens of the cancer cells and/or tissues. In this fashion the homeostatic equilibrium should be restored and would be concomitant with a return to health.

The author also thinks that cancer therapy ought to be performed in small steps and incremental doses. In this fashion, treating with chemo, radio, hormonal and/or immuno therapies will not result in the additional perturbation of the already precariously affected homeostasis of the cancer patient.

Acknowledgments:

These notions stem from studies at McGill University (Genetics), Cornell University & Sloan-Kettering Institute (Immunogenetics) and Rockefeller University. I am deeply grateful to all my professors, physicians, advisors, friends and my family."

Reprinted from 2005 "High, Flat, Down And Back Up Again!"- Alain Amzallag, M.Sc. AuthorHouse, Bloomington, IN 47403- www. authorhouse.com/bookstore pp 109-110.

Addendum II

A Universal Treatment Against cancer

The General Theory of cancer Management [1,2,3,4,5,6] has gone a long way since its conceptualization in 1974. Indeed, the "approaches advocated in Alain Amzallag's theory are presently being used clinically in most cancer treatment centers AND there is a lot of Applied Immunotherapy Research"[7]. Baroukh Hashem.

References:

1 'General Theory of cancer Management'. Copyright © 2010 Alain Amzallag, Montréal. Canada.

2 "High Flat Down And Back Up Again!" "A Guide to Manic-Depressive Illness Copyright © 2005 Alain Amzallag, M.Sc., AuthorHouse, Bloomington IN 47403, U.S.A. www.authorhouse.com/bookstore.

3 "Bipolarité et cancérologie" "Défis et Espoirs" Copyright © 2009 Alain Amzallag, M.Sc., Fondation littéraire Fleur de Lys, Lévis, Québec G6V 2L1 www.manuscritdepot.com.

4 "Anatomy of a vision" "Systems Equilibrium Theory as a General Theory of cancer Management Copyright © 2010 Alain Amzallag, M.Sc., Fondation littéraire Fleur de Lys, Lévis, Québec G6V 2L1 www.manuscritdepot.com.

5 "Réflexions" Copyright ©2012 Alain Amzallag, Ph.D. Fondation littéraire Fleur de Lys, Lévis, Québec G6V 2L1 www.manuscritdepot.com

6 "Reflections" Copyright © 2012 Alain Amzallag, Ph.D. Fondation littéraire Fleur de Lys, Lévis, Québec G6V 2L1 www.manuscritdepot.com

Alain Amzallag – Ph.D.

7 Nicole Beauchemin, Ph.D., Goodman McGill cancer Centre (personal communication, March 21st, 2012).

In memory of:

Monsieur Jacques Abitbol Z"L
Madame Eliane Abitbol-Amzallag Z"L
Mister Terry Fox Z"L
All cancer victims

Note From The Author

Since the age of 13, the author's Bar-Mitzvah in 1962, he obsessed about cancer and the necessity and urgency to find a cure or at least a universal treatment against cancer. In 1974, Alain has a vision of such a universal treatment just prior to undergoing an acute schizoid episode. This vision was subsequently repressed and personal doubts about its applicability in clinical trials abounded in his mind.

Twenty-six years later, the General Theory of cancer Management and the Systems Equilibrium Theory resurfaced (year 2000) in the author's mind as his late mother relapsed during her breast cancer courageous fight. Mme Eliane Abitbol-Amzallag Z"L passed away on March 22nd, 2004. May she rest in peace…

In 2005, Alain published "High, Flat, Down And Back Up Again!" "A Guide to Manic-Depressive Illness", wherein he describes to some extent the main elements of the General Theory of cancer Management. In 2009, Alain Amzallag publishes, this time in French: 'Bipolarité & cancérologie" "Défis & Espoirs".

In 2010, "Anatomy of a vision" is published. In it, the dissection of the vision as conceptualized in 1974 is offered. Describing the genesis of the two theories and the story underlying their discovery, provides insights into Alain Amzallag's thought processes during the Spring of 1974.

These three books attempt to sort out the author's 'bipolar perception', namely; Bipolar Affective Disorder, Type1 and his evolving conviction that the theory has current validity.

From 2005 to 2012, Alain publicized extensively and to the hilt his Theory always seeking feedback from cancer researchers, physicians and oncologists but obtained hardly ever comments from them.

Recently, Alain Amzallag obtained a very important feedback, i.e., a most gratifying reward for his efforts, i.e., the fact that "the approaches advocated in the General Theory of cancer Management are being utilized in the majority of cancer treatment centers AND that there is a lot of research in Applied Immunotherapy". Thank you Nicole…

Alain Amzallag, Ph.D. (ABD)
Montréal, Canada
March 26ᵗʰ, 2012
3 Nissan 5772

A Protocol For Treating Cancers

<u>In memory of</u>:

> Monsieur Jacques Abitbol Z"L
> Madame Eliane Abitbol-Amzallag Z"L
> Mister Terry Fox Z"L
> All cancer victims Z"L

> "We have to beat cancer, all of us, together" – Terry Fox

This protocol for treating cancers advocates using a <u>multi-pronged</u> approach that utilizes, initially, low levels of established therapeutic tools. Specifically, these include the simultaneous use of chemo-, radio-, and hormonal therapies and/or immunological treatments at the onset of cancer therapy.

Then, progressively, doses are increased during intermediary stages of therapy while monitoring the effects of the treatment on cancer cells and/or tissues.

This protocol is intrinsically flexible in nature. It can be custom made for each cancer patient, with the effects on individual patients monitored and adjusted accordingly as strategies and tactics go forward.

Most importantly, this protocol involves an aggressive and multi-<u>pronged</u> attack on cancer: initial, low doses of therapeutic agent(s) are gradually, in discrete increments, followed by increased levels of anti-cancer therapies, until an optimal level is reached. In this way, healthy cells and tissues are not compromised while cancer cells succumb to the <u>synergetic</u> effects of several types of treatments. Once the patient is deemed "cancer-free," a maintenance dose of low-level therapeutic agent(s) helps to prevent a cancer recurrence. Moreover, appropriate diet and exercise then serve to act as a adjunct catalyst for a complete <u>return to health</u>.

Through each phase of this protocol, the types of treatments (chemo-, radio-, hormonal and immunological therapies) are to be used simultaneously.

At each subsequent stage that incorporates incremental small increases of treatment, flexibility is essential as the oncologist decides whether to favour, at any given point in time, one type of therapy over another based on his/her professional experience.

Familial studies have clearly demonstrated that genetic factors are often relevant in regards to the odds of developing cancer. So are carcinogenic chemicals, tumour viruses in lytic or lysogenic cycles, and certain wavelengths of radiation. At the cellular level, these cancer-causing agents initially trigger mutations in the genetic material and transform cells into tumors. Later, these mutated cells are observed to lack "contact inhibition" properties such as are seen in normal tissue during wound healing. The outer cell membranes of cancer cells tend to reflect the presence of abnormal structural and functional protein components. Gene loci such as ER_1PR and HER-2 (code for cell surface receptors) confer highly invasive and metastatic properties to malignant cells. These receptors may be considered as cell surface antigens, which may or not be immunogenic, and which mediate morphogenetic movement (similar to those seen during embryogenesis) in tumor tissue as well as in healthy cells and organisms[1].

The human epidermal growth factor, receptor 2-HER-2, promotes the growth of cancers, most notably breast cancer. The biological therapeutic agents Herceptin® and Tykerb,™ directed specifically against H2R-2[+ve] receptors, have been proved to be very effective on breast cancer cells[5]. Low-dose anti-cancer treatments of cells or tissues that are in their resting phase (S_o) and typically display slow growth and little DNA synthesis or duplication, will probably result in conferring relative hormetic resistance to these cells, as very few mutations will occur under these circumstances. In vitro testing of human tumour cell lines of several tissue types have demonstrated that several hundred chemical and physical stressors appear to trigger the display of hormetic-like biphasic dose responses [3]. However, at low levels of treatment, in vitro tumor cells lines are stimulated to grow and hence will have an increased destruction rate [3] and an even higher one during later incremental increases of the therapeutic agent.

In contradistinction, these biological and chemical molecules, if chemotherapeutic, are toxic to rapidly dividing cells and tissues when administered at high doses from the start, [2,3,4] leading to indiscriminate cellular destruction of both healthy cells (hair follicles, etc.) and cancer cells.

This protocol for treating cancers takes into account both the hormetic and/or the therapeutic aspects of low-dose responses insofar as it advocates using low doses [2,3,4] of anti-cancer agents at the start of cancer treatments. The protocol[2] also recommends combining several different low-dose anti-cancer therapies simultaneously in order to generate synergetic effects [2,3,4] on the cancer while minimizing possible deleterious effects on normal and healthy cells and tissues.

This multi-pronged attack on cancerous cells at low doses, as a first step of treatment, can be considered to be very aggressive because the multiplicity of the simultaneous chemo-, radio- (with several portals), hormonal blocking agents (Tamoxifen), and immunological treatments[2] (Interferon-α, Interleukin-2, monoclonal antibodies, etc.), create a synergetic environment. It stands to reason that this approach will yield improved anti-cancer treatment outcomes.

"Human tumor cell lines commonly display hormetic (biphasic) dose responses" (Calabrese, E.J., 2005)[3] is an in vitro observation that can be extrapolated to also take place in an in vivo scenario. Indeed, low doses of therapeutic physical or environmental stressors are able to distinguish between transformed (cancer) cells and normal healthy cells by targeting rapidly dividing cells. A multiplicity of low-dose therapies[2] in cancer patients will initially result in the preferential elimination (or synergetic effect) of free floating cancer cells that are seeking to establish secondary foci of cancer cells in distant organs (metastasis).

Once these single cells have been eradicated in the patient, increasing the doses of therapeutic agents will lead to combating the spread of neoplasia in the lymphoid system (lymph nodes, spleen, thymus, appendix, etc). The end result would be to circumscribe and contain the primary tumor, which, then and only then, would be ready for surgical removal.

Ideally, at an oncological level blood tests and analyses on cancer patients would be conducted every 15 days, in personalized treatments by low dose multiple therapies, as the best way to follow the progress of the cancer regression[2]. DNA Repair Enzymes would be used to correct mutations in the DNA such as: base (A.G.C.T.) substitutions with base analogs; modifications; deletions; breakage of DNA strands; frame shift mutations; etc.

These mutations are in large measure caused by the oxidation brought about by mutagens in the environment (asbestos, radiation of various wavelengths, DNA and RNA oncogenic viruses, smoke stacks, industrial runoffs, oil spills in oceans, pesticides, etc.), which directly or indirectly mutate the genetic material, i.e., chromosomal DNA.

In the advent that a mutation is not corrected in a timely way, transcription will yield an incorrect messenger-RNA which, in turn, will result in a defective (or no) protein during Translation and ultimately glycosylation, thus altering the structure and/or function of important cell components.

This phenomenon of erroneous protein sequences and glycosylation could be invoked in the context of Tumor Specific Antigens (T.S.A.'s) on cell membranes. If these T.S.A.'s are cryptic, meaning not readily detected by the Immune Surveillance mechanisms (humoral and/or cellular mediated), cancer cells will thrive, ultimately invading neighbouring tissues and colonizing distant organs with metastasis.

It is also possible that T.S.A.'s are present on the outer membranes of single cancer cells or as part of the intercellular matrix which mediates morphogenetic (topology) movement of healthy cells and tissues, as well as in cancerous tissues. This failure of the Immune Surveillance System to detect T.S.A.'s could be construed as being the result of stearic hindrance inherent in abnormal proteins' (Re: mutations) secondary and tertiary structures (di-sulfide bonds).

Theoretical and practical notions in cancer immunotherapy[1] (1974) (2000) (2005) (2009) (2010) (2012) (2014):

In the early 1970's, a prevalent theory about cancer postulated that cancer is an imbalance of the homeostasis of the organism. This author believes that this is still largely true. Indeed, exposure to radiation, chemical mutagens, or oncogenic viruses result in the accumulation of mutations in the DNA sequence, with cancer ensuing. If the DNA repair process and the immune surveillance mechanisms are not able to cope with these mutations past a genetically predetermined threshold, cancer will occur. The mechanism by which the loss of contact inhibition, invasiveness and metastasis operates is at the cell surface level. Cell membrane surface components mediate morphogenesis in the tissues of healthy organisms. In cancer, growth occurs beyond the normal limits, a case of morphogenesis gone awry.

In practical terms, a still untested approach to treat cancer would be to expose cryptic cell surface tumor-specific antigens, derived from cancer cells or tissues, to a variety of mechanical or enzymatic digestion techniques, including cutting into small pieces (mincing), fragmenting with sound waves (sonicating) or enzymatically using pepsin or papain in dissociating the tumor cell membrane while ensuring that the antigenic determinants such as Glycoproteins are not altered or lost of their secondary structure. Then, the resulting preparation would be mixed with adjuvant and administered to the patient. Presumably, the antigenic determinants, previously cryptic, in this self-originating vaccine would become immunogenic and elicit an immune response directed towards the tumor-specific antigens of the cancer cells or tissues. In this fashion, the homeostatic equilibrium would be restored and would be concomitant with a return to health.

References:

1 This section is reprinted from Amzallag Alain © 2005, "High, Flat, Down and Back "Up Again!" "A Guide to Manic-Depressive Illness". AuthorHouse, Bloomington, IN: 2005, pages 17-110.

2- "General Theory of cancer Management" Amzallag Alain Copyright © 2010 Montréal, Canada. Also, in "Reflections" et "Réflexions" Copyrights ©2012 Fondation littéraire Fleur de Lys, Lévis, Québec G6V 2L1 www.manuscritdepot.com.

3"The occurrence of hermetic dose responses in the toxicological literature, the Hormesis data base: an overview" Edward J. Calabrese and Robyn Blain. Toxicology and Applied Pharmacology, Vol 202 (2005) pp 289-301.

4 - "Anatomy of a vision" "Systems Equilibrium Theory as a General Theory of cancer Management" Copyright© 2010 Fondation littéraire Fleur de Lys, Lévis, Québec G6V 2L1 www.manuscritdepot.com

5- National Cancer Institute fact sheet: http://www.cancer.gov/cancertopics/fact sheet/therapy/herceptin

6- Calabrese, E. J. Crit. Rev. Toxicology 2005; 35 (6) 463-582

Being Heard Comforts & Heals Me

TRANLATION FROM FRENCH BY ALAIN AMZALLAG, M.SC.
OCTOBER 24TH, 2015

I like being heard. A number of times in my life I had the impression to be smothered by insolvable problems or to be caught up in vicious catch-22 infernal circles. For a while, feelings of despair and indignity made be believe that I was on the verge of experiencing psychosis. I feel that I have been happier than others to have met at those times individuals who have been able to hear me and free me from the chaos of my feelings. I had the luck to encounter people who could hear more deeply the meaning of what I was saying. These people listened to me without bearing judgement, without affording a diagnosis and neither appreciating nor evaluating me. They have simply listened, clarified what I was saying and answered at every level what I was trying to communicate. I am able to assure you that when you are in such psychic disarray and that someone is really listening to you without bearing judgement and without attempting to influence you, it is really gratifying. Every time it has released the tension that was permeating me. This has enabled me to express the frightening feelings that inhabited me, feelings of culpability and despair, and the confusions that had been my lot in life. When I have been heard and listened to, I become capable of perceiving with a new eye my interior world and move forward. It is surprising to see that the problems that seemed terribly difficult to resolve become easy to understand and decipher when someone hears us, and that situations which seem irremediably confusing become enlightened when someone understands us. I am deeply appreciative of the moments I have met this sensitive, empathic attention that were granted to me.

From: "Liberté pour apprendre"
        de: C.Rodgers, p.222

Ode to my Mom

Born in Azémour, a small village in Central Morocco, my late mother, Mrs. Éliane Amzallag, Z"L, was the youngest of nine children. Several generations have witnessed, in this village, the emergence of scholarly and erudite men (rabbis) and their female equivalent, the *tzadikot* (saintly women). My mother was one such person, whose main intent and purpose in life was to express her joyful kindness to people surrounding her, making them happy in the process. My Mom's predestined name is Frê'ha, a Judeo-Arabic word meaning "Joy". As far back as I can remember, she applied this joy to uplift everyone around her. All my life, she tackled my self esteem problems by encouraging me skillfully and to the hilt.

In 1974, I had my first manic episode while pursuing my graduate studies in New York City and following hospitalization, my health was in shambles. She welcomed me back in her home in Montreal and almost single handedly nursed me back to sanity and well being. She blew a wind of hope that disintegrated my feelings of helplessness. The courage that inspired me led me to start my own family. This tender loving care she provided for over a year, is what almost every mother would do for her child. However, my Mom was a support for me throughout the thirty years of my illness along with the twelve years of her own struggle with a lethal form of breast cancer. What was remarkable about my mom was so that despite the excruciating pain she was enduring, she exercised incredible restraint when I was around so that I would be spared being a witness to her own pain. This was heroic on her part, as her exuding internal fortitude was contagious and did wonders during my faltering moments. Indeed, being afflicted with Bipolar Affective Disorder, Type I, I am extremely sensitive and emotional. During twelve years she hid her pain, but at what cost...

My Mom knew what I wanted to hear, which she did not always tell me; she also knew what I needed to hear, which she delivered readily, providing me with an essential sense of identity and importance in this world. The love in her eyes spread through my chest, my soul, my heart and my mind. Only Mom could make me feel that way, in an instant! As you know, megalomania is a phenomenon often associated with Bipolar Disorder, and this scourge eventually led to my personal bankruptcy. Although my salary was in the six figures, I was always short of cash. My Mom scolded me for spending too much money, but occasionally gave me a $20 bill despite the fact she was living on a pension. This is one of the many examples of the self abnegation she practiced routinely. While her cancer was spreading, she continued to exercise her hospitality duties, as usual. She would host 12 to 15 guest dinners on Jewish holidays such as Passover and Rosh Hashanah. My own family was always invited and very few people were aware of her medical condition because she was so welcoming and cheerful. As a matter of fact, she instructed her immediate family not to divulge her illness to anyone. She wanted to live her life to the fullest until very close to the end. In the face of such unshaken resolve, courage and indomitable morale, my own seasonal anguishes and anxieties quickly dissipated.

When I was irritable, I took refuge at my Mom's home, where I knew I would not be antagonized. She left me alone, and waited until I requested attention. She would then softly allay my fears and calm down my inner demons with her soothing voice. Some may call it babying or excessive tender loving care, but my Mom knew instinctively that the way she acted was in fact "What the doctor ordered". Before cancer struck, Mom, she handled my depressions over the phone, six to eight times a day. Again, with her loving and soothing voice, she would welcome me in her home in the middle of the afternoon for a 2-hour nap. She recognized the importance of sleep in depressed states. My Mom protected my sleep like a watchdog, thus avoiding an upsurge of irritability.

By far, my Mom was the most inspirational figure in my life. She displayed strength, resilience, courage and hope for herself and for her loved ones. She also taught me that in managing my condition I have to make adjustments and personal concessions in order to limit, and build resistance, to internal and external stress.

My Mom was Tall   My Mom stood Tall   My Mom stands Tall

in my heart.

I love you Mom   I miss you Mom

Stigmas And Taboos

Stigmas are the negative thoughts and attitudes that the general population manifests toward mental illnesses. People are sometimes condescending, fearful and unfair (particularly within the job market) to individuals who suffer from mental illness mainly due to ignorance and lack of information about these diseases.

Individuals affected with mental illnesses need, are entitled to, and deserve support from not only their loved ones, but also from the general population. Snide remarks, sneers and tasteless jokes are definitely counterproductive to the healing process and often leave the sufferer with a deeper feeling of rejection and alienation.

Learning about and understanding the origins and cause of the phenomena associated with these illnesses will result in the abating and the erosion of these detrimental stigmas and taboos.

Taboos:

The friends and families of a mentally ill person often experience a sense of helplessness, shame and fear because of the stigmas associated with these illnesses, because of their own lack of knowledge and because of the worrisome fear that they themselves may one day be affected. As a result of these factors, the friends and loved ones of a mentally ill person tend to be secretive, going to great lengths to hide the illness from others. This often results in a lack of the support that is desperately needed by their loved one. In their shame, they will shield themselves and their loved one from groups and from gossip that are perceived as detrimental. Also, family and friends often withdraw from the affected individual out of their fear and misunderstanding of the uncharacteristic, emotional outbursts that can accompany these diseases.

"STIGMAS AND TABOOS FEED ON EACH OTHER, CREATING A "CATCH 22" SITUATION (VICIOUS CIRCLE). IF ONE ATTEMPTS TO DISSIPATE AND REDUCE THESE TWO TANDEM PHENOMENA, THEIR IMPACT ON THE MENTALLY ILL AND THEIR FAMILIES CAN BE LESSENED."

We believe it is time that we start to put these stigmas and taboos behind us. We must realize that everyone has something in his or her lives to deal with, that everyone is "disabled" in some sense of the word. We believe that people, especially those suffering from mental illnesses, should become aware of their strengths and their positive attributes and focus on these. If family and friends support this process, recovery for the mentally ill person may be less fraught with difficulty. When people are afraid to open up, they miss the opportunity for support in all its ways and yet another vicious circle gains momentum.

It is ironic that anyone should associate stigmas with mental illness at all since the mode of hereditary transmission is not yet completely understood. This means that anyone is susceptible to becoming mentally ill! Indeed, epidemiological and statistical studies have shown that around twenty percent of the population, at some point in their lifetime, will suffer from some form of mental disorder. It is true that anyone who has had a relative who has suffered from mental illness is "at risk" for developing some forms of the condition themselves. Yet, just how much risk is impossible to determine or predict. We do know that genes are involved with these illnesses. It may be important to note here that ancestors, while they may have suffered from mental illness, were often undiagnosed and just labeled "eccentric".

Many individuals identified as mentally ill have conveyed to others, in writing, the story of their journey within and through a mental illness to a place of functionality. These individuals have written about managing their condition in order to become, or remain, operational. In addition to being a form of therapy, writing from our own perspectives and perceptions can very often be cathartic, allowing healing to take place. These authors encourage this process, as it benefits not only the writer, but may also benefit others making or watching such a journey. If you seek to publish it, who knows how many your story may inspire!

Families who are in the midst of the hurt and turmoil caused, in large part, by the silent aspect of the taboo should seek to obtain information from the many organizations who offer information and support; the Canadian Mental Health Association, the Mood Disorders Society/Association of Canada, and a number of other organizations within North America. These organizations have been established to inform, support and also to create awareness and understanding of mental illnesses.

A person suffering from a mood disorder should not be subject to judgment or condemnation by any other member of society, including those closest to them. Rather, they need people to talk to and to support them during this time of deep personal crisis.

As knowledge and understanding erode these stigmas, it is our hope and belief that taboos will slowly release their stifling stranglehold, permitting the normalization and acceptance between an "affected family" and the "world outside".

LET US ALL PRAY FOR HUMANENESS TOWARD THE MENTAL WORLD

Alain Amzallag
Montréal, Canada

E-mail : <u>alainamzallag@bell.net</u>
Site Web : <u>www.alainamzallag.com</u>

Observations By Alain Amzallag August 1St, 2007

I think I am emotionally disturbed, perturbed…

- - I get angry at people close to me (related) very easily, I scream in moments of excessive stress…
- I cry with an extreme ease when I am upset by a sad situation…
- My mood changes from one minute to the next…
- I have a hard time watching local & world news on television…
- Some songs make me cry…
- Some songs make me sod (sangloter…)
- Gory pictures make me sick and afraid…
- Some elements of paranoia inhabit me…
- I am either extremely happy (pushing the limits…) or very sad…
- I can sometimes be obsessive and sometimes compulsive (timing of phone calls) …
- For no obvious or apparent reason, often, tears appear in my eyes…
- I am struggling with bipolarity-Je me débas avec la Bipolarité

Depression

The Symptoms of Depression are:

1 - Depressed Mood.
2 - Loss of Interest / Pleasure.
3 - Decreased ability to think clearly / Concentrate.
4 - Low Self-Esteem / Guilt Feelings
5 - Recurrent thought of Death and suicide.
6 - Loss of Energy and Fatigue.
7 - Loss or Gain of appetite / Change in weight.
8 - Insomnia or sleeping too much.
9 - Too much or too little energy.

Associated Symptoms:

A- Anxiety.
B- Social withdrawal.

The criteria for Major Depression are:

1 - Five out of nine symptoms (described above) for two weeks or more.
2 - Symptoms occurring all the time.
3 - Severe consequences.
4 - Not related to substance abuse (i.e. alcohol) or illness (i.e. Thyroid).
5 - Must be distinguished from mourning.

Please, if you have 5 out of these 9 symptoms, you are most likely undergoing a Major Depression and therefore you should contact your physician **IMMEDIATELY**. Antidepressants will be prescribed to you in order to restore your normal mood.

* Note: These antidepressants may create some unpleasant side effects. However, these are generally temporary- Please, give these Medications a chance to help you.

** Note: If you suffer from Major Depression, please, do not feel singled out as 20% of the world population will at one point or another have Mood Difficulties.

<u>*Your health is precious to you and to us*</u>.

Alain Amzallag, M.Sc.
May 20th, 2006
Montréal

Dealing With Mental Illness

The first step in dealing with mental illness is to realize and <u>acknowledge</u> that something, somehow, is wrong with your emotional and thought processes and abilities. The second step is to seek help -- by visiting your family doctor -- and to consider what colleagues, friends and members of your family tell you; they will almost certainly have noticed some changes in your personality, temperament and character.

If your troubles are due to depression, it may advisable to take a trip south to a sunny spot at a more hospitable latitude. If the trip cannot be taken, light therapy is an option and must be considered: being exposed to 10,000 LUX every morning for 30 minutes is an efficient way to fight depression and lift the spirits. The author is a firm believer in the benefits and therapeutic value of light therapy.

Alternatively, your general practitioner and/or your psychiatrist can prescribe anti-depressants to help you, your mood, and lower your anxiety and suffering. However, antidepressants can have unwanted effects. These depend on the patient's physiological and neurological reactions to the medication. However, one generally adjusts to these symptoms after a few weeks.

An important third step in combating mental illness is to select a psychiatrist you are compatible with, whom you trust and with whom you feel free to confide every symptom and feeling, the changes that occur with each tweak of medication, and the stresses of your day-to-day life.

The fourth step and, in the author's mind, the most important one, is to face mental illness head-on and to muster the courage to figure out what is wrong, and take the first steps in learning to manage the illness. Once this decision is made, the patient and his/her psychiatrist can decide on a regimen of medication and therapy and adjust their levels until the optimal doses are reached so that the patient can become once again functional and flourishing.

Moreover, once the optimal level of medications and stress-avoidance steps are achieved, monitoring the course of treatment by the patient becomes the prime component in living a healthy and productive life.

If there happens to be a loss of contact with reality, meaning a manic (psychotic) episode, hospitalization for a few weeks becomes mandatory, with a variety of steps pit onto place for for rehabilitation.

As for hypomania, the ease of conceptualization, and the artistic and musical inspirations are pleasurable. However, one must be careful, as the ugly head of the mania awaits.

Be well and be good…!

Alain Abraham Amzallag, M.Sc.
September 18th, 2010
Montreal, Canada

References:

1 – Copyright © *2009*.Amzallag, Alain, M.Sc. *Bipolarité & Cancérologie. Défis & Espoirs*: Fondation littéraire Fleur de Lys, Levis, Qué *G6V 2L1*.

2- *Copyrigh*t © *2005*. Amzallag, Alain, M.Sc. *High, Flat, Down And Back Up Again! A Guide to Manic-Depressive Illness. AuthorHouse, Bloomington, IN 47403*

Appendix – Psychiatry – Think Tank

Article For Brainstorm 2014-2015

Mental Illness & Homelessness:

Are most of the Homeless people mentally ill...?

If we consider that, <u>at least</u>, for Bipolar Affective Disorder (BAD), the locus carrying the gene(s) for BAD is linked (co-inherited) to genes responsible for addiction to drugs and alcohol, then, the answer to the question asked above is a **"prudent yes"**...

Most of us have witnessed the emotionally erratic behaviour of the homeless individuals as well as the display of symptoms during a psychotic episode. It is at that exact moment that first responders should seize the opportunity and use, in a gentle way, their persuasive talents to bring the homeless to an emergency room of a Hospital with a psychiatric ward. This has to be done skilfully as homeless people are known to dislike psychiatric wards.

<u>Note</u>: Once the homeless patient is given a bed on the psych ward, it is important that during the rehabilitation, the patient is assigned a social worker in order to address the patient's living quarter's problems. These social workers assigned to the rehabilitation (from a psychotic episode; drug addiction; alcoholism and a predilection to life in the streets) of homeless persons must be able to inspire trust as well as guide their patients towards self esteem workshops and accompany them through the difficult initial stages of drug and alcohol weaning of their deep addictions. These social workers should be kind, convincing as well as assertive in their dealings with homeless people...

But why are the homeless se reluctant to being hospitalized and receive treatment (medications and/or psychotherapy)...? Perhaps life in the streets enables them to escape the harsh reality of a "normal life" with all the responsibilities and efforts it entails.

Also, maybe living in the streets takes them away from prior experiences of physical and/or psychological abuse. Moreover, living in the streets confers them with the seemingly desirable sensation of freedom... To regain a normal life's serenity involves giving up this freedom, the "highs" of drug usage and alcohol consumption.

Alain Amzallag, Ph.D (ABD)
alainamzallag@bell.net
www.alainamzallag.com

"Improving Relations Between Police Forces And Mentally Ill Individuals In Canada"

By Alain A. Amzallag, M.Sc.
Montréal, Canada

Need for this project:

The improvement of relations between police forces, emergency services, security agents and correctional facility personnel and people suffering from mental health issues is necessary and essential.

Sometimes, signs of distress which manifest themselves by unusual behaviours in persons in a psychotic state (Bipolarity and/or Schizophrenia or deep depression with risk of suicide) escape the attention of emergency personnel or can be construed as verbal abuse which could turn into verbal and/or physical violence…

Firstly; it is of paramount importance to attempt to ***calm down*** the affected and erratic individual.

Secondly, cleverly and skilfully accompany or transport by ambulance towards a hospital which is equipped to handle persons in psychotic state, i.e., with a psychiatrist on call and a psych ward in case an hospitalisation proves to be necessary.

Important items:

Members of police forces should acquaint themselves with the results of the Commission on Mental Health of Canada, i.e., Michel Kirby's vision and report; and let this superb piece of work be inspirational during encounters with people with mental illnesses; for example: the homeless who often struggle with psychological and / or psychiatric difficulties that render them addicted to drugs and alcohol. Please, visit: the Canadian Association for Mental Health: www.cmha.ca and the Mood Disorders Association of Ontario: www.mooddisorders.ca.

Several Mental Health Associations in Montréal provide valuable information on mental health issues on their Web Site as well as in their Newsletters. These are, "Revivre": www.revivre.org"; Amiquébec": www.amiquebec.org ; Amitié / Friendship" www.assobenevoleamitie.cam.org ; and the Association of Québec Psychiatrists: www.ampq.org.

The various police forces in Canada ought to familiarise themselves with the different diagnostics, signs and symptoms of the different mental illnesses, so that better preparation and ability to perform their duty optimally will result in avoiding worst case scenarios. It is, according to the author, desirable that the general population, as well as mentally distressed persons, perceive, view and consider police forces as representing benevolent authorities seeking order and harmony in society.

In conclusion, our law makers should promote legislations that will make impossible the acquisition of weapons of any kind by people with a psychological or psychiatric instability.

Alain Amzallag, M.Sc. is a free lance writer and lecturer on mental health and issues – to contact the author: www.alainamzallag.com or alainamzallag@ bell.net.

Introduction

After writing and publishing three books (2005)[1] (2009)[3] (2014)[8] on Bipolarity, type 1, based on personal experience and which are largely autobiographical, the author, Alain Amzallag decides to solicit the contribution and/or the comments of some twenty or so Mental Health professionals with regard to finding solutions to pressing mental health issues... Alain Amzallag, the moderator of this Think Tank selected these professionals whom he knows well enough to believe that, for all intents and purposes, their goals and objectives are to diminish the suffering of mentally ill patients and to do everything in their power to enlighten where darkness once prevailed... As well, these individuals wish to convey their assistance through their knowledge during the process of abating the demons of psychotic breaks...

In 1974, Alain A., then a graduate student, was inspired to develop the concept of Systemic Equilibrium which proved to be useful in cancer management as well as in the management of several other chronic diseases (2010)[4]. Mental illness can be construed as a chronic disease as once a major depression and/or a psychotic episode has taken place; the most the patient can hope for is to overcome the symptoms by taking medications (antidepressants; mood stabilisers; neuroleptics) and psychotherapy with the desire to reach full functionality...

Alain A. would like to open a discussion on the application of the Systems Equilibrium concept to understand and manage mental illnesses.

Systems Equilibrium Theory:

In the same manner as electrons in orbit and protons in the nucleus mutually maintain their respective positions, and as gravitational forces in operation in nature keep objects and planets in place relative to each other (with or without apparent motion), it is evident that a uniform, intrinsic and harmonious equilibrium exists and operates in the Universe, and that it maintains thorough stability. Although the word *systems* used in this title, addresses the conceptualization of these equilibriums separately, it is obvious that these systems are interdependent and if one is faulty, others can go awry (environment, disease [mental illness], war, famine, and so forth). In view of these postulated systems equilibriums, one ought to effect change in small increments in order not to disturb the equilibriums, so that they may continue to enjoy their buffered flexibility. If the equilibrium of a system is disrupted, it follows that reparative doses, actions or treatments should be applied gradually in small increasing steps....

Just as in several multi-factorial and late-onset genes, in mental illness nature (genes) interact with nurture (environment) to generate symptoms of depression and/or psychosis. A fruitful approach could be to find ways to use elements of nurture (stressors) to ***buffer*** the expression of genetic predisposition (nature). For example, when mental illness predisposition in children and/or teenagers has been noticed or diagnosed, one could do the following: A) Avoid high to extreme stress or B) Strengthen gradually resistance to stress... A) & B) could be done simultaneously, gradually and progressively, in small increments...

The Systems Equilibrium concept[4] is applicable to the treatment of symptoms associated with some mental illnesses. Mentally ill patients have an imbalance; either chemical and/or physiological at the neuronal level. Moods are affected by the level of neurotransmitters such as: Serotonin, Dopamine and Noradrenalin, as well as the consumption of certain foods. The relative and proportional amounts of these neurotransmitters are keys to determining whether one is happy, sad or just content as well as the various shades in between...

[1] Under the heading of Mood Stabilizers, the following is a presentation based on an article by Isabelle Artus and sections summarized by Didier Chos, on how nutritional elements can help regulate variations in mood;

"Dopamine, Serotonin and Noradrenalin are neurotransmitters that jointly regulate mood, energy level, harmony and indeed determine our "Happiness". When the level of serotonin is insufficient, the mood dips rapidly, sometimes leading to aggressive behavior; this is followed by sleep disorders, bad mood and sometimes depression. Serotonin is labeled the "Good Humour Hormone". A precursor to both serotonin and dopamine is the amino acid Tryptophan and seeking foods that contain Tryptophan is necessary to maintain a stable level of these two neurotransmitters. Starchy foods, fish, rice etc. contain Tryptophan. However, too much simple sugars, and/or stimulants like nicotine or caffeine reduce the serotonin content in the brain. This happens because your system depletes your serotonin reserve a while after you ingest these substances. You ingest these substances; you get a high and your mood crashes a few hours later; thus the addiction cycle continues. REMINDER: balanced blood sugars levels promote balanced mood. To achieve a balanced mood, you need enough serotonin producing protein and insulin balancing polyunsaturated "good" fats." Now, a deficiency in dopamine leads to difficulties in concentrating and to a loss in motivation, dopamine is geared to stimulate the heart and general metabolism. Noradrenalin increases motivation and energy levels and acts as an anti depressant as well". "A non-essential amino acid L-Tyrosine found in seafood, cheese, milk and eggs, is a precursor to noradrenalin and dopamine, adequate energy level and a good dose of optimism, the aforementioned foodstuff should be eaten".

Warning: It is of paramount importance to realize that the aforementioned nutritional tips cannot replace prescribed medications, but they can enhance their efficacy.

Identifying major problems:

1) Suicides caused by bullying
2) Drug and alcohol addictions
3) Improving relations between police forces and mentally ill persons
4) Preventing possession of weapons of any kind by mentally ill persons

5) Supporting legislation for achieving # 4)
6) Stigmas in the work place must be denounced and dissipated
7) Taboos within families must be eliminated proactively and progressively
8) Search and glorify the success stories of the Clara Hughes of this world
9) Creation of sheltered work places to positively favor mentally ill persons

Please, feel free to tackle one of the above or other mental health associated problems by suggesting and expressing ideas and replying to this e-mail address: alainamzallag@bell.net

Bibliography:

1 "High, Flat, Down and Back Up Again!" "A Guide to Manic-Depressive Illness" Copyright © 2005 Alain Amzallag, M.Sc. AuthorHouse, Bloomington, Indiana 47403 USA www.authorhouse.com/bookstore (discontinued)

3 "Bipolarité et Cancérologie" "Défis et Espoirs" Copyright © 2009 Alain Amzallag, M.Sc. Fondation littéraire Fleur de Lys, Lévis, (Québec) G6V 1A8 www.manuscritdepot.com

4 "Anatomy of a vision" "Systems Equilibrium Theory as a General Theory of cancer Management and other Chronic Diseases" Copyright © 2010 Alain Amzallag, M.Sc. Fondation littéraire Fleur de Lys, Lévis, (Québec) G6V 1A8 www.manuscritdepot.com

5 "Réflexions" (Santé Mentale / Prose Profonde / Théorie de Gérance du cancer) Copyright © 2012 Alain Amzallag, M.Sc. Fondation littéraire Fleur de Lys, Lévis, (Québec) G6V 1A6 www.manuscritdepot.com

6 "Reflections" (Mental Health / Deep Prose / Cancer Management Theory) Copyright © 2012 Alain Amzallag, M.Sc. Fondation littéraire Fleur de Lys, Lévis, (Québec) G6V 1A6 www.manuscritdepot.com

If you live in Canada, these six books written by Alain Amzallag can be purchased by sending an e-mail to the author: <u>alainamzallag@bell.net</u> Upon receipt of your cheque, the book(s) will be posted to your address.

Si vous vivez au Canada, ces six livres écrits par Alain Amzallag peuvent être achetés en expédiant un courriel à l'auteur: <u>alainamzallag@bell.net</u> Sur reception de votre chèque, le (s) livre (s) vous seront expédiés par la poste.

Mental Health Think Tank

<u>MENTAL HEALTH & GENE THERAPY:</u>

The ever quickening advances of science made possible by the success of the Human Genome Project will also soon let us see the essences of mental disease. Only after we understand them at the genetic level can we rationally seek out appropriate therapies for such illnesses as schizophrenia and bipolar disease. James D. Watson – *Nobel Prize laureate.*

With the advent of the Human Genome Project, it is possible nowadays to sequence completely, and in a few days, the genes that comprise an individual's genetic makeup. This opens the door to "Gene Therapy". In early 2014, in an In-Vitro Fertilization experiment in mice, scientists were able to create an offspring without an undesirable gene. It is noteworthy that men and mice have 97% of their genetic material with an identical sequence. In a few years, it will be possible to achieve gene therapy with humans and in the process create designer babies and individuals. However, for gene therapy in humans to be beneficial to humanity, it must be accompanied by the most stringent ethical restrictions so as to preclude the resurgence of the ugly head of Eugenics. Alain Amzallag, Ph.D. (ABD)

Reprinted from; "High, Flat, Down And Back Up Again!" "Insights on Bipolarity" "Challenges & Hopes" (Revised) (2014) Alain Amzallag AuthorHouse, Bloomington Indiana 47403

<u>MENTAL HEALTH & MARIJUANA:</u>

BIPOLAR PERCEPTION:

Concerning soft narcotics such as marijuana, hashish and kef, the inhaling of smoke derived from these substances leads to a psychotropic distortion of the sounds and sights of the surroundings. Moreover, an emotional surge yields a "high", the intensity of which is contingent upon the potency and the purity of the drug.

We know that people affected with Bipolar Affective Disorder are generally very sensitive to practically everything. The author believes that the hereditary component of the Bipolar Disorder causes a predisposition to this mental condition by diminishing the baseline ability of the affected individual to endure stress.

Recently, it has been established that excessive usage of drugs may trigger mental illness in individuals and in particular those with a predisposition.

This triggering took place in this author's life in Fall 1973…

It all fits: the affected person has a genetic predisposition which renders him or her unable to withstand too much stress and therefore, upon consumption of the drugs, the nervous system is weakened and major depression and/or a manic episode ensue.

This scenario is congruent with the occurrence of post-partum depressions whereby the tremendous pain and stress of birthing sometimes leads to post-partum psychosis.

There seem to be an increase in spirituality in the mind and the words of persons undergoing a psychotic episode whether they had one or a few…

In my case, 1974 was the start of a 30 year intensive study of the Bible…

Since 1973, I have not consumed any drugs or alcohol. Interestingly, for the last 30 years or so, Nature in all its magnificence and forms (Human Beings, Animals, Vegetal & Mineral formations), has filled my heart, my soul and my mind with its inherent beauty and these feelings were accompanied with incomparable and sometimes ecstatic delight…

This having been said, are the drugs still having an effect on me after 45 years? If this were the case, this delayed action phenomenon could account for visions and hallucinations occurring in some normal and some mentally troubled individuals who have consumed the weed...

On the chemical standpoint, such occurrences could be explained by postulating that the psycho-active molecules in drugs bind permanently to the neuronal cell surface receptors and that although it would be to a reduced extent, the effect would be for all intents and purposes irreversible. In addition, it has been established by neurophysiologists that marijuana most probably destroys neurons---- Good luck pot-heads!

Alain Amzallag, M.Sc.
September 2007

Reprinted from "Reflections" (2012) Alain Amzallag Fondation littéraire Fleur de Lys, Lévis, (Québec) G6V 1A8

-=-=-=-=-

December, 2014, 4Th Communication Mental Health Think Tank

"The Canadian government's stance on Marijuana (2014) must be applauded as well as its efforts to warn the general public of the dangers of smoking it..." Alain A.

Clinical depression and attempted suicide

Deep depressions or Major depressions are often triggered in individuals with a proclivity to mental illnesses by emotional or chemical stressors. Depressions and/or psychotic breaks can also be caused by soft drug over usage and/or very often the root causes of depressions is a love / hate relationship spiraling down to an intense hellish level and sometimes involves a love betrayal.

In general, individuals have a threshold (genetically coded in their DNA) of stress resistance capacity, which, if lowered by mental illness and/or combined with smoking potent marijuana and/or being in a painful love/ hate relationship will eventually develop a Major depression. When the symptoms of Major depression include bouts of anxiety and/or anguish, this depression is regarded as a Clinical depression which requires medical and/or psychiatric attention. Tale-tale signs of a deteriorating Clinical depression are when the individual runs in his head different scenarios as to how ending their own life as the pain endured seems to be unbearable and it seems that the only way to stop the pain would be to commit suicide. Some categories of individuals are prone to Deep Depressions and because of their mental health issues may attempt to end their lives; Teenagers coming from dysfunctional homes, War Veterans and Homeless people are all at risk for attempted suicide.

Antidepressants, Zoo-Therapy & Light Therapy are excellent tools to address this Clinical depression. However, psychiatric hospitalization may become necessary; mainly if fleeting thoughts of suicide go though the person's mind and these fleeting thoughts of suicide must be addressed immediately with a mental health professional that will help the patient decipher the reason(s) for the dark thoughts.

Ironically, one of the ways that can lighten one's depression's exacting symptoms would be to find again "True Love" while one is revisiting one's previous amorous relationship(s). In the 60's, the moderator read a sign on the front of a fixer's shop in Cape Cod: "We repair everything except a broken heart"... Retrospectively, a broken heart can be mended (the moderator contends) by basking in the comforting warmth and brightness of a lover's embrace.

Also, another way to lessen the suffering caused by one's mental state is to rely on Faith & Belief in the Creative Entity and look for and find spiritual sustenance, through study and practice, in the Scriptures. A variety of Religions & Spiritualities lend themselves quite well for that purpose, i.e., Judaism, Zen Buddhism, and so on.

Basically, a deeply depressed individual, with the help of a Mental Health professional, should aim at restoring the balance, the equilibrium between his/her Spirit, his/her Emotions & his/her mental state. This can be achieved with proper nutrition, physical exercise and taking religiously the prescribed medications as well as seeking assistance from available resources such as: Psychiatrists, Psychologists, Psychiatric Nurses, Social Workers, self-esteem and laughing workshops, and most importantly communicate your feelings with people around you and/or express or pour out the contents of your soul through Art and / or Music (listening, performing, composing) and / or writing Prose and / or Poetry. G-d bless...

List Of Publications By Alain Amzallag, M.sc., Ph.d.

1 - "Genetic Fine Structure of the Leucine Operon of Escherichia coli K-12". J.M. SOMERS, A. AMZALLAG, AND R.B. MIDDLETON. JOURNAL OF BACTERIOLOGY, Mar, 1973, p. 1268-1272

2 - "A study of mouse alloantigens by indirect immunofluorescence" Alain Amzallag (1974) Masters of Science Thesis. Cornell University Graduate School of Medical Sciences / Sloan-Kettering Division, NYC, N.Y. 10021

3 - "High, Flat, Down And Back Up Again !" "A Guide to Manic-Depressive Illness". © 2005 Alain Amzallag, M.Sc., AuthorHouse, Bloomington IN 47403, U.S.A. www.authorhouse.com/bookstore

4 - "The Art, the Sport and the Science of Salesmanship" "Giving of oneself without expecting returns", © 2006 Alain Amzallag, M.Sc., AuthorHouse, Bloomington IN 47403, U.S.A. www.authorhouse.com/bookstore

5 - "Bipolarité et Cancérologie" "Défis et Espoirs", © 2009 Alain Amzallag, M.Sc., Fondation littéraire Fleur de Lys, Lévis, Québec G6V 2L1 www.manuscritdepot.com
Page personnelle d'Alain Amzallag dédiée à ce livre sur le site de la Fondation littéraire Fleur de Lys : http://www.manuscritdepot.com/a.alain-amzallag.1.htm

6 - « Anatomy of a vision » « Systems Equilibrium Theory as a General Theory for Cancer Management and Other Chronic Diseases" © 2010 Alain Amzallag, M.Sc., Fondation littéraire Fleur de Lys, Lévis, Québec G6V 2L1 www.manuscritdepot.com
Page personnelle d'Alain Amzallag dédiée à ce livre sur le site de la Fondation littéraire Fleur de Lys: http://www.manuscritdepot.com/a.alain-amzallag.2.htm

7 - « Pensées d'Avi ben Mordékhaï » Copyright © 2010 Alain Amzallag, M.Sc. Fondation littéraire Fleur de Lys, Lévis, Québec, G6V 2L1 www.manuscritdepot.com

Page personnelle d'Alain Amzallag dédiée à ce livre sur le site de la Fondation littéraire Fleur de Lys : http://www.manuscritdepot.com/a. alain-amzallag.3.htm

8 - « Réflexions » Copyright © 2012 Alain Amzallag, Ph.D. (ABD) Fondation littéraire Fleur de Lys, Lévis, Québec G6V 2L1 www. manuscritdepot.com *Page personnelle d'Alain Amzallag dédiée à ce livre sur le site de la Fondation littéraire Fleur de Lys :* http://www. manuscritdepot.com/a.alain-amzallag.4.1.htm

9 - « Reflections » Copyright © 2012 Alain Amzallag, Ph.D. (ABD) Fondation littéraire Fleur de Lys, Lévis, Québec, G6V 2L1 www. manuscritdepot.com *Page personnelle d'Alain Amzallag dédiée à ce livre sur le site de la Fondation littéraire Fleur de Lys :* http://www. manuscritdepot.com/a.alain-amzallag.4.2.htm

10 -« Sea Storm » « Insights on Bipolarity » « Challenges & Hopes » Copyright © 2013 Alain Amzallag, M.Sc. Fondation littéraire Fleur de Lys, Lévis, (Québec) G6V 2L1 www.manuscritdepot.com *Page personnelle d'Alain Amzallag dédiée a ce livre sur le site de la Fondation littéraire Fleur de Lys* http://www.manuscritdepot.com/a. alain-amzallag.6.htm

11 -« Spirit of Sales » « Giving of Yourself without expecting returns » Copyright © 2014 Alain amzallag, Ph.D. (ABD) Fondation littéraire Fleur de Lys Lévis, (Québec) G6V 2L1 www. manuscritdepot.com
Page personnelle d'Alain Amzallag dédiée à ce livre sur le site de la Fondation littéraire Fleur de Lys http://www.manuscritdepot.com/a. alain-amzallag.7.htm

12 -« High, Flat, Down And Back Up Again! » (Revised) Copyright ©2014 Alain Amzallag, Ph.D. (ABD) « Insights on Bipolarity » « Challenges and Hopes » AuthorHouse, Bloomington, Indiana 47403 www.authorhouse.com/bookstore www. manuscritdepot.com

13 -"MEDS & REMEDIES" (2018) Copyright © Alain Amzallag, Ph.D. AuthorHouse, Bloomington Indiana 47403 USA www. authorhouse.com / bookstore.

14 -ARTICLES IMPORTANTS RÉDIGÉS ET PUBLIÉS PAR ALAIN AMZALLAG:

IMPORTANT ARTICLES WRITEN AND PUBLISHED BY ALAIN AMZALLAG:

A- Stigmas & Taboos -Copyright © 2010 Alain Amzallag All rights reserved Equilink: Ontario Moods Disorders Association Newsletter

B- "General Theory of cancer Management" Copyright © (2010) Alain Amzallag, Ph.D. All rights reserved

C- Taming depression Copyright.© Alain Amzallag, Ph.D. (2008) All rights reserved

D- Bipolar stress Copyright © Alain Amzallag Ph.D. (2007) All rights reserved

E- Bipolar perception Copyright © Alain Amzallag, Ph.D. (2007) All rights reserved.

F- Expression Copyright © Alain Amzallag (2007) All rights reserved

Acknowledgements

FRIENDS FOR LIFE:

- Serge Segal: long time reliable & self abnegating friend.
- Bob Shiley: most trustworthy & trusted friend.
- Sarita Benchimol: most supportive scientific & social friend
- the multitasking dynamo.
- Claudine Suissa: One huge giving heart and cute to boot.
- Rav Abraham Abitbol: Talmudic genius & poet.

Jean Coutu

I am truly grateful to Emad Gabra, Ph; Stephan Dolarian, Ph.; Carla Chirinian, Ph.; Mekouar Amina, Ph., Haiduc Corrina, Ph. Dabo Makan, Ph, for their constant and precise, personalised and conscientious work of verifying (scrutinizing) the contents of my dispels. Thank you again. Please don't tell the M.D.'s that I value your experience more than I do theirs. AND THAT'S THE TRUTH!

Bob Shiley, your support in good as well as in tough times has proven to be invaluable. Spiritually, we are one. Indeed, often we communicate by E.S.P., and I apologize for not letting you know that my silence was due to a lengthy hospitalization. As you know Toronto is only a five-hour drive from Montreal, in which you and Anne have a standing invitation to my home.

St. Mary's Hospital:

The author is truly grateful to Dr Dominique Ferrarotto. M.D. for modifying the time at which the Neuroleptic Orap (Pimozide) is prescribed to Alain A. at some point during his 46 day-hospitalization on the 8th floor of St. Mary's Hospital. From bedtime uptake, with the undesirable side effect of a very deep sleep facilitating dypsiuria, Dr. Ferratto decided that A.A.A. will take the Orap early in the morning. This led to a spectacular improvement of the situation, i.e., Alain's sleep was not as deep, his days were more awake and full of energy and very importantly, incontinence disappeared totally and finally.

Soeur Marie-Andrée, M.D.

Je vous suis reconnaissant pour l'excellence des soins personalisés et attentionnés que vous avez octroyés à mon égard. J'ai eu le privilège d'entrevoir un aspect de votre âme que perçue comme bonne, belle et généreuse. Que D'ieu vous bénisse et vous protège afin que vous puissiez continuer à ramener des enfants de D'ieu troublés et égarés dans notre monde réel…Amen…!

Kathy and Bobby, Executive Directors of the Jewish Community Foundation of Montreal have always been fans of the outcome of the author's literary efforts, while participating with sponsorship, they also provided judicious advice and incalculable empathy that spurred A.A.A. to surmount many obstacles he encountered…

To Contact Author:

alainamzallag@bell.net

Personal Trilingual Web site:

(English / Français / Español)

www.alainamzallag.com

Printed in the United States
By Bookmasters

Printed in the United States
By Bookmasters